A THYROID RESET DIET COOKBOOK

Energize Your Thyroid

Nourishing Recipes for a Balanced Life

ROLAND BLESSING

TABLE OF CONTENT

INTRODUCTION 9

CHAPTER 1 14

Understanding Thyroid Health 14

The Thyroid and Its Crucial Role in the Body: A Symphony of Balance 16

Navigating the Terrain of Common Thyroid Disorders: Unraveling the Intricacies ...19

Hypothyroidism 20

The Slumbering Thyroid 20

Hyperthyroidism 20

The Accelerated Symphony 20

Hashimoto's Thyroiditis 21

A Symphony of Autoimmunity 21

Graves' Disease 21

The Hyperactive Crescendo 21

Thyroid Nodules 22

A Subtle Dissonance 22

Navigating the Path Forward 22

Harmony on the Plate: The Intricate Connection Between Diet and Thyroid Function ...23

1. Iodine: The Conductor's Baton 23

2. Selenium: 24

3. Nutrient-Dense Composition: The Musical Score of Well-Being 24

4. Cruciferous Vegetables: A Thoughtful Crescendo 25

5. Hydration: The Fluidity of Thyroid Support 25

CHAPTER 2 26

The Thyroid Reset Approach: A Symphony of Renewal for Vibrant Health 26

What is a Thyroid Reset Diet? 29

Principles and Goals of the Thyroid Reset Diet 30

Principles: 30

Goals: 32

Benefits of Resetting Your Thyroid 33

Getting Started with the Thyroid Reset 36

1. Consultation with Healthcare Professional: 37

2. Comprehensive Thyroid Panel: 37

3. Set Realistic Expectations: 37

4. Educate Yourself: 38

5. Cleanse Your Pantry: 38

6. Begin with Nutrient-Rich Foods: 38

7. Mindful Meal Planning: 38

8. Hydration and Lifestyle Adjustments: 39

9. Regular Monitoring: 39

10. Celebrate Small Wins: 39

CHAPTER 3 40

Foundations of Thyroid-Friendly Eating 40

Iodine-Rich Foods 40

Selenium SPage | 4ources 42

Zinc-Packed Options 45

Antioxidant-Rich Superfoods 48

Harnessing the Power of Berries 51

CHAPTER 4 55

Resetting Your Plate - Recipes for Thyroid Support 55

1.   55

Breakfast Boosters for Thyroid Reset Diet: Fueling Your Day with Nutrient-Rich Morning Choices 59

1. Oatmeal Power Bowl: 60

2. Protein-Packed Smoothie: 60

Tips for Breakfast Success: 64

Quinoa and Berry Breakfast Bowl 65

Energizing Lunch Ideas for Thyroid Health 67

1. Salmon and Quinoa Salad: 67

2. Sweet Potato and Chickpea Buddha Bowl: 68

3. Turkey and Vegetable Stir-Fry: 69

4. Spinach and Berry Salad with Chicken: 69

5. Mango and Shrimp Quinoa Bowl: 70

6. Vegetarian Lentil Soup: 71

Tips for Thyroid-Friendly Lunches: 71

Nourishing Dinner Delights for Thyroid Reset 72

1. Grilled Salmon with Roasted Vegetables: 72

2. Turmeric Chickpea Stew: 73

3. Chicken and Vegetable Stir-Fry: 74

4. Mushroom and Spinach Quinoa Risotto: 74

5. Shrimp and Asparagus Stir-Fry: 75

6. Lentil and Vegetable Curry: 76

Tips for Thyroid-Supportive Dinners: 76

Seaweed-Wrapped Salmon Rolls for Thyroid Reset Diet 77

Prepare Salmon Slices: 78

Assemble Ingredients: 79

Rolling Technique: 79

Slice into Rolls: 79

Garnish and Serve: 79

Dipping Sauce: 79

Snacks and Sides for Thyroid Reset Diet 81

Snacks: 81

Greek Yogurt Parfait: 81

Roasted Chickpeas: 82

Seaweed Snacks: 82

Nuts and Seeds Mix: 82

Dark Chocolate and Almonds: 83

Sides: 83

☐   Quinoa Salad: 83

☐   Steamed Broccoli with Tahini: 83

☐   Sweet Potato Wedges: 83

☐   Cauliflower Hummus: 83

Sautéed Spinach with Garlic: 84

Quinoa Stuffed Bell Peppers: 84

Tips for Snacks and Sides on a Thyroid Reset Diet: 84

Balance Macronutrients: 84

Portion Control: 84

Incorporate Iodine-Rich Foods: 84

Hydration: 84

Whole, Minimally Processed Foods: 85

Thyroid-Friendly Smoothie for Resetting Your Diet 86

Spinach or Kale: 86

Berries (Blueberries, Strawberries 86

Greek Yogurt: 86

Chia Seeds or Flaxseeds: 86

Coconut Water or Almond Milk: 87

Banana: 87

Brazil Nuts: 87

Iodine-Rich Foods (optional): 87

Tips for a Thyroid-Friendly Smoothie: 88

Balance Macros 88

Incorporate Iodine-Rich Ingredients 88

Limit Added Sugars: 88

Variety is Key: 89

Hydrate: 89

Consult with a Professional: 89

CHAPTER 5 90

Crafting Thyroid-Supportive Meal Plans 90

Key Components: 90

Iodine-Rich Foods: 90

Selenium Sources: 90

Omega-3 Fatty Acids: 90

Fruits and Vegetables: 91

Protein-Rich Foods:..91

Whole Grains: 91

Healthy Fats: 91

Weekly Meal Planning Guide:..91

Sample Weekly Meal Plan:..94

Tuesday:94

Wednesday:..95

Thursday:..95

Friday: 95

Tips for Success: 96

Smart Substitutions and Ingredient Swaps for Thyroid Reset Diet: 97

Tips for Success: 100

Elevating Flavors with Herbs and Spices for Thyroid Reset Diet: 101

1. Turmeric:...102

2. Ginger: 102

3. Rosemary: 102

4. Cinnamon: 102

Tips for Incorporating Herbs and Spices:..104

CHAPTER 6..106

Beyond the Plate - Lifestyle Tips for Thyroid Health...106

Exercise Strategies for Thyroid Function 106

1. Cardiovascular Exercise: 106

2. Strength Training:..107

3. Interval Training:..107

4. Yoga and Stretching: 107

5. Outdoor Activities: 108

6. Mind-Body Practices: 108

7. Consistency is Key: 108

8. Listen to Your Body: 109

9. Warm-Up and Cool Down: 109

The Role of Yoga and Meditation for Thyroid Reset...110

1. Stress Reduction: 110

2. Balancing Hormones: 110

3. Improved Sleep Quality: 111

4. Enhanced Circulation: 111

5. Mind-Body Connection: 111

6. Reduced Inflammation: 112

7. Energy Regulation: 112

9. Improved Mental Health: 113

10. Holistic Approach: 113

Incorporating Yoga and Meditation: 114

Stress Management Techniques for Thyroid Reset 115

1. Mindfulness Meditation: 115

2. Deep Breathing Exercises: 115

3. Progressive Muscle Relaxation (PMR): 116

4. Guided Imagery and Visualization: 116

5. Yoga and Tai Chi: 116

6. Aromatherapy: 116

7. Journaling: 117

8. Nature Walks: 117

9. Social Connections: 117

Prioritizing Quality Sleep for Thyroid Support 118

Why Quality Sleep Matters for Thyroid Health 118

Tips for Prioritizing Quality Sleep: 120

Conclusion 122

Nurturing Your Thyroid Journey 122

APPENDIX A: THYROID-FRIENDLY INGREDIENT LIST 1257.   Essential   Nutrients   for   Thyroid   Health:
.... 127

APPENDIX B: QUICK REFERENCE COOKING TIPS 131

INTRODUCTION

Sarah was a very vibrant young lady, full of life until she fell ill. Despite her vibrant spirit and zest for life, Sarah found herself trapped in a cycle of fatigue, unexplained weight gain, and a persistent feeling of sluggishness. Concerned, she sought the guidance of medical professionals who diagnosed her with an underactive thyroid, a condition that explained her symptoms.

Determined to regain control of her health, Sarah began researching ways to support her thyroid naturally.

In her quest for knowledge, she stumbled upon the concept of the Thyroid Reset Diet. Intrigued, she delved into the principles behind this transformative approach.

The Thyroid Reset Diet emphasized nourishing the body with specific nutrients essential for optimal thyroid function. Armed with this newfound understanding, Sarah set out to overhaul her eating habits.

She bid farewell to processed foods and embraced a diet rich in iodine, selenium, and nutrient-dense whole foods. Her kitchen became a haven of colorful fruits, leafy greens, and lean proteins, each bite carefully chosen to fuel her body and support her thyroid.

The mornings transformed into a ritual of vitality for Sarah. She started her day with a nutrient-packed smoothie, blending together berries, spinach, and a sprinkle of chia seeds. This breakfast not only energized her but also kick-started her metabolism, setting a positive tone for the rest of the day.

Lunch and dinner became opportunities for culinary exploration. Sarah experimented with recipes designed to incorporate thyroid-friendly ingredients.

From salmon and avocado salads to quinoa bowls teeming with colorful vegetables, her meals were not only a treat for her taste buds but also a symphony of nutrients supporting her thyroid health.

Alongside her dietary changes, Sarah embraced lifestyle adjustments. She incorporated regular exercise, focusing on activities that promoted thyroid function. Yoga and meditation became integral parts of her routine, offering both physical and mental rejuvenation.

As the weeks passed, Sarah noticed subtle yet significant changes. Her energy levels surged, the unexplained weight gain began to reverse, and a newfound clarity replaced the mental fog that had clouded her mind.

Encouraged by these positive shifts, she continued to follow the Thyroid Reset Diet with dedication and commitment.

One day, during a follow-up appointment with her healthcare provider, Sarah received uplifting news.

Her thyroid function had improved, and the once-subdued gland was now operating within normal parameters. The journey of thyroid reset, fueled by a nourishing diet and mindful living, had transformed Sarah's health.

With a revitalized spirit, Sarah continued to embrace the Thyroid Reset Diet as a way of life.

Her story became an inspiration for others facing similar challenges, proving that with the right knowledge, dedication, and a nourishing approach, one could reset not just their thyroid but also their entire well-being.

And so, Sarah's journey became a beacon of hope for those seeking a path to thyroid wellness through the transformative power of the right diet.

Welcome to a transformative journey towards revitalizing your well-being through the power of the Thyroid Reset Diet. Your thyroid, a small but mighty gland nestled in your neck, plays a pivotal role in your overall health.

Yet, too often, its significance is overlooked. If you've been grappling with fatigue, weight fluctuations, or a sense of unexplained imbalance, your thyroid might be quietly pleading for attention.

The Thyroid Reset Diet is not just a collection of recipes; it's a holistic approach to nourishing your body, resetting your metabolism, and reclaiming the energy and vitality that may have eluded you. This isn't a one-size-fits-all solution; it's a tailored roadmap to support thyroid health, recognizing that each individual's journey is unique.

In this book, we'll unravel the mysteries of thyroid function, explore the intricate dance between your diet and thyroid wellness, and empower you with practical tools to make informed choices.

Whether you're facing thyroid challenges or simply seeking to proactively boost your metabolic resilience, the Thyroid Reset Diet is a powerful ally in your pursuit of optimal health.

Prepare to embark on a culinary adventure filled with nutrient-rich, delicious recipes designed to nourish your body and support thyroid function. But it's not just about what's on your plate; it's a comprehensive lifestyle shift encompassing mindful practices, stress management, and tailored exercises to create a harmonious environment for your thyroid to thrive.

As you delve into these pages, remember: this is more than a cookbook; it's an invitation to rediscover the vitality within you. Embrace the Thyroid Reset Diet with enthusiasm, commitment, and an open heart, and let the journey towards a revitalized you begin.

Here's to a vibrant life fueled by the nourishing embrace of the Thyroid Reset Diet.

CHAPTER 1

Understanding Thyroid Health

In the intricate symphony of the human body, the thyroid gland emerges as a conductor, orchestrating a myriad of functions that influence overall well-being.

 Nestled in the neck, this butterfly-shaped gland holds the key to metabolism, energy regulation, and the delicate equilibrium of various bodily systems.

To comprehend thyroid health is to appreciate the multifaceted role this unassuming gland plays. At its core, the thyroid produces hormones—thyroxine (T4) and triiodothyronine (T3)—that influence metabolism and energy production.

Like messengers, these hormones traverse the bloodstream, reaching every cell in the body to ensure proper functioning.

At the heart of the thyroid's prowess lie thyroxine (T4) and triiodothyronine (T3) – two hormonal marvels that act as messengers of metabolic command.

These hormones are not mere spectators; they are conductors, wielding influence over the body's metabolism and energy production.

Much like a conductor directs an orchestra, the thyroid hormones navigate the bloodstream, weaving through the intricate channels to reach every cell with precise instructions for optimal functioning.

Picture these hormones as ethereal messengers, dancing through the arteries and veins, navigating the bloodstream with purpose. Their destination? Every nook and cranny of the body, ensuring that the wheels of cellular activity turn smoothly.

From the tips of our fingers to the depths of our organs, the thyroid hormones whisper the secrets of equilibrium, signaling cells to produce energy and maintain a delicate balance.

In the intricate ballet of metabolism, the thyroid's role is nothing short of noble. It not only dictates the speed at which our body utilizes energy but also regulates temperature, heart rate, and the efficiency of our organs. A harmonious interplay of T4 and T3 ensures that the body's engine runs at the optimal pace, fostering a state of vibrant health.

To comprehend thyroid health is to stand in awe of the thyroid's multifaceted mastery. It's an acknowledgment that within this unassuming gland resides a powerhouse, a guardian of balance, and a weaver of vitality. As we delve into the complexities of thyroid function, let us appreciate the elegance with which these hormones traverse the bloodstream, orchestrating a symphony of well-being that resonates at the cellular level.

The Thyroid and Its Crucial Role in the Body: A Symphony of Balance

The thyroid, a small, butterfly-shaped gland nestled in the neck, might be unassuming in size, but its influence on the intricate dance of human physiology is nothing short of profound. Like a skilled conductor directing a symphony, the thyroid orchestrates a myriad of bodily functions, ensuring harmony and balance throughout the entire ensemble.

1. Regulating the Metabolic Symphony: At the core of the thyroid's role lies its ability to regulate metabolism, the body's complex process of converting food into energy.

The thyroid achieves this by producing two vital hormones: thyroxine (T4) and triiodothyronine (T3). These hormones act as metabolic conductors, influencing how quickly cells convert nutrients into energy. In essence, the thyroid sets the tempo for the metabolic symphony, ensuring a finely tuned performance.

2. Temperature Control: The Thyroid's Conductor Baton: Beyond metabolism, the thyroid also plays a pivotal role in regulating body temperature. Much like a thermostat, it adjusts the internal heat to maintain a constant and optimal temperature. When the body needs to generate more heat, the thyroid hormones signal an increase in metabolic activity, and conversely, when less heat is required, metabolic activity decreases.

This elegant dance ensures the body operates within a narrow temperature range essential for optimal function.

3. A Guardian of Growth and Development: The thyroid extends its influence to the intricate processes of growth and development, especially in children. Proper thyroid function is crucial for the development of the brain and the skeletal system. Inadequate thyroid hormones during critical periods can lead to developmental challenges, making the thyroid a guardian of not just metabolic health but also the unfolding journey of human growth.

4. Maintaining Cardiovascular Harmony: The thyroid's impact extends to the cardiovascular system, where it helps regulate heart rate and blood pressure. Thyroid hormones influence the responsiveness of blood vessels and the heart to ensure a steady flow of blood throughout the body. This orchestration is essential for

maintaining cardiovascular health and supporting the delivery of oxygen and nutrients to all tissues.

5. A Balancing Act- The Thyroid's Symphony of Well-Being: In essence, the thyroid is the conductor of a complex symphony, directing the rhythms of metabolism, temperature, growth, and cardiovascular function. Its influence permeates every cell, and its absence or imbalance can lead to a discordant tune in the orchestra of human health.

Understanding and nurturing the thyroid is, therefore, not just an exploration of a gland; it is a journey into the heart of bodily harmony and balance, where the thyroid's symphony of well-being resonates with precision and grace.

Navigating the Terrain of Common Thyroid Disorders: Unraveling the Intricacies

In the delicate orchestration of thyroid function, a misstep can lead to a discordant tune in the symphony of health. Common thyroid disorders, affecting millions worldwide, cast a spotlight on the gland's vulnerability and its profound impact on well-being. Let's delve into the intricacies of these disorders, understanding the nuances that shape their manifestation.

Hypothyroidism

The Slumbering Thyroid

Hypothyroidism, an underactive thyroid, occurs when the gland fails to produce sufficient thyroid hormones (T3 and T4). This deficiency can cast a pervasive shadow over vitality, manifesting in symptoms such as fatigue, weight gain, cold sensitivity, and cognitive sluggishness. The orchestra of metabolism, in this case, plays at a subdued tempo, leading to a sense of lethargy and unexplained weight fluctuations.

Hyperthyroidism

The Accelerated Symphony

On the opposite end of the spectrum lies hyperthyroidism, an overactive thyroid condition. Here, the gland produces an excess of thyroid hormones, setting the metabolic symphony on a frenetic pace. Symptoms may include loss of weight, increased heart rate, anxiety or fear, and heat intolerance. The body, akin to an orchestra racing through a piece, experiences a heightened state of activity that can lead to unintended consequences.

Hashimoto's Thyroiditis

A Symphony of Autoimmunity

Hashimoto's thyroiditis, an autoimmune disorder, unfolds when the body's immune system mistakenly attacks the thyroid tissue. This relentless assault can gradually impair the thyroid's ability to produce hormones, eventually leading to hypothyroidism.

Hashimoto's often manifests with symptoms similar to those of hypothyroidism, emphasizing the complex interplay between the immune system and thyroid health.

Graves' Disease

The Hyperactive Crescendo

In contrast, Graves' disease, another autoimmune disorder, prompts the thyroid to overproduce hormones. This heightened activity can result in hyperthyroidism, characterized by symptoms such as weight loss, bulging eyes (exophthalmos), and an accelerated heartbeat. Graves' disease exemplifies the intricate nature of autoimmune conditions, where the body's defenses turn against its own tissues.

Thyroid Nodules

A Subtle Dissonance

Thyroid nodules, though often benign, can introduce a subtle dissonance to the thyroid's symphony. These small lumps or growths on the thyroid can lead to the overproduction of hormones (hyperthyroidism) or, conversely, cause hypothyroidism if the nodules disrupt the gland's normal function. While most nodules are harmless, some may warrant further investigation to rule out malignancy.

Navigating the Path Forward

Understanding common thyroid disorders is akin to deciphering the musical score of the body's intricate symphony. As individuals navigate the terrain of thyroid health, early detection, medical guidance, and a holistic approach to well-being become essential notes in orchestrating a harmonious tune. By embracing awareness and fostering a partnership with healthcare professionals, individuals can navigate the complexities of thyroid disorders and strive for a life in harmony with their well-being.

Harmony on the Plate: The Intricate Connection Between Diet and Thyroid Function

In the intricate dance of human physiology, the relationship between diet and thyroid function emerges as a crucial symphony, where the notes on the plate resonate deeply within the thyroid's delicate chambers. Understanding this intricate connection unveils a pathway not only to nourishment but also to the harmonious well-being of one of the body's most influential conductors.

1. Iodine: The Conductor's Baton

At the heart of thyroid health lies iodine, an essential trace element often likened to the conductor's baton orchestrating the thyroid's symphony. Iodine is a very important component in the synthesis of thyroid hormones, T3 and T4. Without sufficient iodine, the thyroid's ability to produce these vital hormones is compromised, potentially leading to hypothyroidism. Seaweed, iodized salt, and seafood stand as rich sources, ensuring the conductor's baton is wielded with precision.

2. Selenium: The Harmony Enhancer

Selenium, a powerful antioxidant, emerges as a harmony enhancer in the diet-thyroid connection. This trace mineral aids in the conversion of T4 (thyroxine) to the active T3 (triiodothyronine) hormone. A deficiency in selenium may hinder this conversion process, influencing thyroid function. Brazil nuts, sunflower seeds, and fish contribute to the symphony of selenium, ensuring the thyroid's harmonious function.

3. Nutrient-Dense Composition: The Musical Score of Well-Being

The composition of one's diet plays a pivotal role in supporting overall thyroid function. A diet rich in nutrient-dense foods such as fruits, vegetables, lean proteins, and whole grains provides the essential vitamins and minerals that contribute to the thyroid's vitality. These foods serve as the musical score, with each nutrient playing a unique note in the harmonious melody of well-being.

4. Cruciferous Vegetables: A Thoughtful Crescendo

While cruciferous vegetables like broccoli, cauliflower, and cabbage are nutrient-rich powerhouses, their consumption requires a thoughtful crescendo. These vegetables contain compounds known as goitrogens, which, in excess, can interfere with iodine uptake by the thyroid. Cooking these vegetables and balancing their intake with iodine-rich foods allows for a harmonious integration into the thyroid's symphony.

5. Hydration: The Fluidity of Thyroid Support

Amidst the dietary notes, hydration stands as a key component in maintaining thyroid support. A well-hydrated body ensures the smooth flow of nutrients, allowing the thyroid's symphony to resonate with fluidity. Water becomes the conductor's baton, facilitating the seamless performance of the thyroid's vital functions.

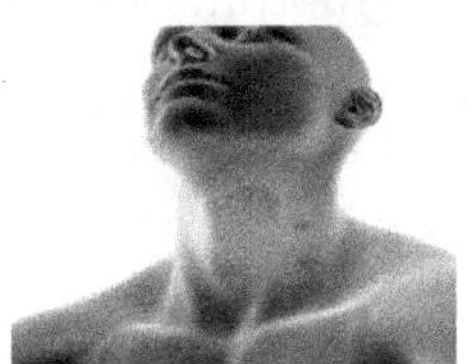

CHAPTER 2

The Thyroid Reset Approach: A Symphony of Renewal for Vibrant Health

In the realm of wellness, the Thyroid Reset Approach emerges as a transformative melody, offering individuals a harmonious journey toward revitalizing thyroid health.

Rooted in the synergy of mindful nutrition, lifestyle adjustments, and a commitment to well-being, this approach orchestrates a symphony of renewal for those seeking to rekindle the vitality within.

At its essence, the Thyroid Reset Approach embodies a philosophy of balance and nourishment.

It acknowledges the intricate interplay between diet, lifestyle, and thyroid function, recognizing that each element contributes to the symphony of well-being.

The approach aims not merely to address symptoms but to reset the foundation, fostering a holistic environment where the thyroid thrives.

Central to the Thyroid Reset Approach is the art of nourishment through thyroid-friendly foods. This includes incorporating nutrient-dense choices rich in iodine, selenium, and essential vitamins.

Berries, leafy greens, lean proteins, and omega-3 fatty acids become the notes in this symphony, contributing to the renewal of the thyroid's vital functions.

Meal planning takes center stage, guided by a thoughtful orchestration of thyroid-supportive ingredients.

The Thyroid Reset Approach provides a blueprint for crafting balanced, delicious meals that cater to the unique needs of thyroid health. A weekly dance of flavors and nutrients ensures a consistent and nourishing melody for the thyroid's renewal.

Beyond the plate, the Thyroid Reset Approach extends its influence to lifestyle factors. Exercise becomes a tailored movement, designed to support thyroid function without inducing stress. Stress management techniques, including mindfulness and relaxation practices, play a pivotal role in maintaining the symphony of hormonal balance.

Quality sleep becomes the restful interlude, allowing the thyroid to rejuvenate and renew its vital functions.

Acknowledging the uniqueness of each individual's journey, the Thyroid Reset Approach encourages personalized care and monitoring.

Regular check-ins with healthcare professionals, understanding one's body signals, and adapting the approach based on individual responses create a dynamic and responsive melody for thyroid health.

The Thyroid Reset Approach is not a quick fix but a journey toward lasting well-being. It embraces the idea that true harmony arises when the mind, body, and spirit are in sync. As individuals embark on this transformative journey, they are invited to savor the symphony of renewal, fostering a profound connection with their thyroid health and overall vitality.

In the ongoing symphony of renewal, the Thyroid Reset Approach stands as a conductor, guiding individuals towards a vibrant and harmonious existence.

By embracing the melody of mindful nourishment, purposeful movement, and holistic well-being, individuals find themselves in tune with the renewal of their thyroid health and the rediscovery of the vitality that resides within.

What is a Thyroid Reset Diet?

A Thyroid Reset Diet is a targeted nutritional approach aimed at restoring and optimizing thyroid function. Focused on nutrient-dense foods, it emphasizes essential elements like iodine and selenium crucial for thyroid health.

Incorporating superfoods, mindful cooking, and balanced meal plans, the diet seeks to create an environment that supports the thyroid's vital role in metabolism and overall well-being. It often integrates lifestyle factors like tailored exercise and stress management for a holistic approach to thyroid health.

The goal is to reset and rejuvenate the thyroid, promoting a symphony of vitality in the body.

The Thyroid Reset Diet is not a one-size-fits-all solution; it encourages individualization based on responses and ongoing monitoring with healthcare professionals.

By embracing this approach, individuals embark on a journey to harmonize their diet, lifestyle, and thyroid function, unlocking renewed energy, balance, and overall wellness.

A Thyroid Reset Diet is a targeted nutritional approach aimed at restoring and optimizing thyroid function. Focused on nutrient-dense foods, it emphasizes essential elements like iodine and selenium crucial for thyroid health.

Incorporating superfoods, mindful cooking, and balanced meal plans, the diet seeks to create an environment that supports the thyroid's vital role in metabolism and overall well-being. It often integrates lifestyle factors like tailored exercise and stress management for a holistic approach to thyroid health. The goal is to reset

Principles and Goals of the Thyroid Reset Diet

The Thyroid Reset Diet is grounded in a set of principles and goals crafted to guide individuals on a transformative journey toward optimal thyroid health. Understanding these principles and goals is key to unlocking the full potential of this holistic approach.

Principles:

1. Nutrient Density: Prioritizing foods rich in essential nutrients, such as iodine and selenium, that are vital for thyroid function. This principle underscores the importance of whole, minimally processed foods for overall well-being.

2. Balanced Macronutrients: Ensuring a harmonious mix of proteins, healthy fats, and complex carbohydrates in each meal. This principle promotes sustained energy, supports metabolic function, and contributes to a balanced nutritional profile.

3. Mindful Cooking: Embracing cooking techniques that preserve the nutritional integrity of foods. This principle encourages methods that enhance rather than diminish the thyroid-supportive properties of ingredients.

4. Superfoods Integration: Incorporating superfoods like berries, leafy greens, and nutrient-rich options known for their positive impact on thyroid health. This principle adds a layer of vibrancy to the diet, enhancing its nourishing properties.

5. Individualization: Recognizing the uniqueness of each individual's body and responses to dietary changes. This

principle encourages personalized adjustments, fostering a tailored approach to the Thyroid Reset Diet.

Goals:

1. Thyroid Restoration: The primary goal is to restore and optimize thyroid function. Achieving this involves providing the thyroid with the essential nutrients it needs, promoting a balanced hormonal environment, and supporting metabolic processes.

2. Energy Revitalization: Rekindling energy levels by nourishing the body with foods that contribute to sustained vitality. The Thyroid Reset Diet aims to lift the veil of fatigue, providing a renewed sense of vigor and well-being.

3. Weight Management: Striving for a healthy weight balance by supporting metabolic function. The diet aims to address fluctuations in weight that may be associated with thyroid disorders, promoting a sustainable and balanced approach.

4. Symptom Alleviation: Mitigating common symptoms of thyroid disorders such as fatigue, cognitive fog, and temperature sensitivity. The goal is to enhance overall

quality of life by alleviating the impact of thyroid-related symptoms.

5. Holistic Wellness: Fostering a holistic sense of well-being that extends beyond nutrition. The Thyroid Reset Diet integrates lifestyle factors like tailored exercise, stress management, and adequate sleep to promote comprehensive health.

6.Long-Term Health: Establishing sustainable dietary and lifestyle habits for long-term health. The goal is not just a temporary reset but a lasting transformation that supports ongoing thyroid health and overall wellness.

Understanding and aligning with these principles and goals empowers individuals to embark on a purposeful Thyroid Reset Diet journey, cultivating a symphony of vitality and balance in their lives and rejuvenate the thyroid, promoting a symphony of vitality in the body.

Benefits of Resetting Your Thyroid

Embarking on the journey of resetting your thyroid can unfold a cascade of transformative benefits, touching not only the intricate symphony of thyroid function but resonating throughout your entire well-being. Here are the key advantages of resetting your thyroid:

1. Enhanced Energy Levels: Balancing thyroid function can alleviate fatigue and lethargy, unlocking a renewed and sustainable wellspring of energy. Individuals often report increased vitality and improved endurance throughout daily activities.

2. Metabolic Harmony: Resetting the thyroid supports metabolic processes, promoting a healthy weight balance and fostering a more efficient utilization of nutrients. Achieving metabolic harmony can contribute to better weight management and a sense of overall wellness.

3. Improved Mental Clarity: Balancing thyroid hormones positively impacts cognitive function, alleviating brain fog and promoting mental clarity. Individuals often experience enhanced focus, concentration, and cognitive sharpness.

4. Mood Stabilization: Thyroid health is closely linked to mood regulation. Resetting the thyroid can contribute to emotional well-being and mood stability.

Individuals may notice a positive impact on their outlook, reducing feelings of anxiety or irritability.

5. Hormonal Balance: Optimal thyroid function influences the balance of other hormones in the body. Resetting the thyroid can contribute to a more harmonious hormonal environment. Improved hormonal balance may lead to benefits such as stabilized menstrual cycles and reproductive health.

6. Restored Sleep Patterns: Thyroid imbalances can disrupt sleep patterns. Resetting the thyroid often results in improved sleep quality and a more restful night.

Individuals may experience a more consistent sleep routine, promoting overall health and well-being.

7. Vibrant Skin, Hair, and Nails: Thyroid health is reflected in the condition of the skin, hair, and nails. Resetting the thyroid can contribute to a more vibrant and healthy appearance. Individuals may notice improvements in skin texture, hair strength, and nail health.

8. Increased Resilience to Stress: Balancing thyroid function supports the body's stress response. Resetting the thyroid can enhance resilience to stressors, both physical and emotional.

Individuals may find themselves better equipped to cope with life's challenges.

9. Long-Term Health and Disease Prevention: A well-functioning thyroid is integral to overall health. Resetting the thyroid contributes to a foundation of well-being that may help prevent future health complications. Individuals may experience a reduced risk of conditions associated with thyroid imbalances.

10. Enhanced Quality of Life: Perhaps the most significant benefit is an overall improvement in quality of life. Resetting the thyroid fosters, a sense of vitality, balance, and well-being that permeates every aspect of daily living. Individuals often report a greater enjoyment of life, increased motivation, and a positive outlook on the future.

As you embark on the journey of resetting your thyroid, these benefits paint a compelling picture of the positive impact on both your thyroid health and your holistic well-being. Each step toward thyroid balance is a step toward a more vibrant and fulfilling life.

Getting Started with the Thyroid Reset

Getting started with the Thyroid Reset is a purposeful initiation into a journey of well-being and vitality. Here are key steps to kick start your Thyroid Reset:

1. Consultation with Healthcare Professional: Begin with a consultation with a healthcare professional, preferably one well-versed in thyroid health.

Discuss symptoms, concerns, and your intention to reset your thyroid for personalized guidance.

2. Comprehensive Thyroid Panel: Request a comprehensive thyroid panel to assess levels of thyroid-stimulating hormone (TSH), T3, T4, and thyroid antibodies. This baseline evaluation provides insights into your current thyroid status.

3. Set Realistic Expectations: Establish realistic expectations for your Thyroid Reset journey. Understand that it's a gradual process, and improvements may take time. Patience and consistency are key elements in achieving sustainable results.

4. Educate Yourself: Invest time in understanding the principles of the Thyroid Reset, including the role of nutrition, lifestyle, and the interconnectedness of thyroid function.

Equip yourself with knowledge to make informed decisions on dietary and lifestyle changes.

5. Cleanse Your Pantry: Conduct a pantry cleanse, removing processed foods, excessive sugars, and items high in unhealthy fats. Stock up on thyroid-friendly foods, including lean proteins, fruits, vegetables, and whole grains.

6. Begin with Nutrient-Rich Foods: Prioritize nutrient-dense foods rich in iodine, selenium, and essential vitamins. Incorporate thyroid-friendly superfoods such as berries, leafy greens, and lean proteins into your meals.

7. Mindful Meal Planning: Initiate mindful meal planning to ensure a balanced intake of macronutrients and a variety of nutrients. Experiment with thyroid-supportive recipes that align with the principles of the Thyroid Reset.

8. Hydration and Lifestyle Adjustments:

Prioritize hydration, a fundamental aspect of thyroid support. Ensure an adequate intake of water throughout the day. Begin integrating lifestyle adjustments, such as tailored exercises, stress management techniques, and sufficient sleep.

9. Regular Monitoring: Establish a schedule for regular monitoring of your thyroid function. Periodic check-ins with healthcare professionals allow for adjustments based on your progress.

Use blood tests and physical indicators to track improvements and adjust your Thyroid Reset accordingly.

10. Celebrate Small Wins: Acknowledge and celebrate small wins along the way. Whether it's increased energy levels, improved sleep, or other positive changes, each step is a victory. Cultivate a positive spirit and focus on the progress made.

CHAPTER 3

Foundations of Thyroid-Friendly Eating

Thyroid-friendly eating involves adopting a balanced and nutrient-dense diet to support optimal thyroid function. The thyroid, a crucial gland in the endocrine system, plays a key role in regulating metabolism, energy production, and overall well-being. Here are some foundational principles for thyroid-friendly eating:

Iodine-Rich Foods

Iodine is a crucial trace element that plays a fundamental role in the synthesis of thyroid hormones, which are essential for regulating metabolism and supporting overall growth and development. Including iodine-rich foods in your diet can help ensure an adequate supply of this essential nutrient. Here are some foods that are good sources of iodine:

- Seaweed: Seaweed, such as nori, kelp, and dulse, is among the richest sources of iodine. It's commonly used in Asian cuisine and can be incorporated into salads, soups, or used as a wrap.

- Fish: Fish, particularly saltwater fish, is a good source of iodine. Examples include cod, tuna, shrimp, and haddock. Fish can be a versatile and nutritious addition to your diet.

- Dairy Products: Dairy foods, including milk, yogurt, and cheese, are reliable sources of iodine. Choosing iodized salt for cooking or seasoning can further enhance iodine intake.

- Iodized Salt: Iodized salt is a simple and effective way to ensure sufficient iodine intake. It is regular table salt fortified with iodine, and it can be used in cooking or as a seasoning.

- Eggs: Eggs contain a moderate amount of iodine, and they are a versatile ingredient that can be incorporated into various dishes for added nutrition.

- Shellfish: Shellfish, such as shrimp, oysters, and mussels, are rich sources of iodine. Including these in your diet provides a flavorful and nutrient-dense option.

- Iodine-Fortified Foods: Some foods, especially processed foods like bread and cereals, may be fortified with iodine. Checking food labels can help identify products that contribute to iodine intake.

- Turkey and Chicken: Poultry, such as turkey and chicken, contains iodine and can be included in a well-balanced diet for a diverse nutrient profile.

It's important to strike a balance when it comes to iodine intake, as excessive consumption can also have negative effects on thyroid function.

The recommended daily intake of iodine varies based on factors such as age, sex, and pregnancy status.

If you have specific concerns about your iodine levels or thyroid health, consulting with a healthcare professional or a registered dietitian is advisable to ensure personalized and accurate guidance.

Selenium Sources

Selenium is an essential mineral that plays a critical role in various bodily functions, including supporting the immune system and aiding in the conversion of thyroid hormones. Including selenium-rich foods in your diet can help maintain adequate selenium levels. Here are some common sources of selenium:

- Brazil Nuts: Brazil nuts are rice in selenium. However, it's important to consume them in moderation due to their exceptionally high selenium content. Just a few nuts can provide the recommended daily intake.

- Seafood: Fish and shellfish are excellent sources of selenium. Tuna, halibut, sardines, shrimp, and crab are examples of selenium-rich seafood.

- Meat: Various meats, including beef, pork, lamb, and poultry, contain selenium. Lean cuts of meat can be incorporated into a balanced diet for selenium intake.

- Sunflower Seeds: Sunflower seeds are a convenient and tasty snack that also provides selenium. They can be enjoyed with salads, yogurt, or enjoyed on their own.

- Whole Grains: Whole grains, such as brown rice, quinoa, and oats, contain selenium. These grains offer not only selenium but also fiber and other essential nutrients.

- Dairy Products: Dairy foods like milk, cheese, and yogurt contribute to selenium intake. Including a variety of dairy products in your diet can support overall nutritional needs.

- Eggs: Eggs, particularly the egg yolk, contain selenium. Eggs are versatile and rich in nutrient and can be included in various dishes.

- Legumes: Legumes, including lentils, chickpeas, and black beans, provide a moderate amount of selenium along with other essential nutrients.

- Brazilian Nuts: Other nuts, such as cashews and almonds, also contain selenium, although in smaller amounts compared to Brazil nuts.

- Mushrooms: Mushrooms, such as shiitake and button, contain selenium. Including a variety of mushrooms in your diet can contribute to overall selenium intake.

It's important to note that the selenium content in plant-based foods depends on the selenium content of the soil in which they are grown. While selenium is vital for health, excessive intake can lead to adverse effects.

As with any nutrient, maintaining a balanced and varied diet is key. If you have specific concerns about selenium levels or dietary choices, consulting with a healthcare professional or a registered dietitian can provide personalized guidance.

Zinc-Packed Options

Zinc is a crucial mineral that plays a vital role in various bodily functions, including immune function, wound healing, and DNA synthesis. Including zinc-packed foods in your diet is essential for maintaining optimal health. Below are some amazing sources of zinc:

- Meat: Red meat, particularly beef and lamb, is one of the best sources of zinc. These meats provide a highly absorbable form of zinc, making them valuable contributors to daily intake.
- Shellfish: Shellfish, such as oysters, crab, and lobster, are rich in zinc. Oysters, in particular, are known for their exceptionally high zinc content.

- Poultry: Chicken and turkey are good sources of zinc. Include lean cuts of poultry in your diet for a healthy dose of this essential mineral.

- Nuts and Seeds: Various nuts and seeds are packed with zinc. Pumpkin seeds (Pepitas), cashews, and almonds are excellent choices to incorporate into your snacks or meals.

- Legumes: Legumes, including chickpeas, lentils, and beans, provide a plant-based source of zinc. These foods are not only rich in zinc but also offer fiber and other nutrients.

- Dairy Products: Dairy foods such as milk, cheese, and yogurt contain zinc. Go for low-fat or no-fat options to limit too much fat intake.

- Eggs: Eggs, particularly the egg yolk, contain zinc. Eggs are a versatile food that can be included in various dishes for added nutrition.

- Whole Grains: Whole grains like quinoa, wheat, and oats contain zinc. Including a variety of whole grains in your diet contributes not only to zinc intake but also to overall nutritional balance.

- Dark Chocolate: Dark chocolate, in moderation, can be a tasty source of zinc. Go for chocolate with a high cocoa content for maximum benefits.

- Fortified Foods: Some foods, such as certain breakfast cereals, are fortified with zinc. Checking food labels can help identify products that contribute to zinc intake.

- Vegetables: Certain vegetables, such as mushrooms and spinach, contain moderate amounts of zinc. Including a variety of vegetables in your diet adds not only zinc but also other essential nutrients.

Maintaining an adequate intake of zinc is essential for overall health, but it's important not to exceed recommended levels, as excessive zinc intake can have adverse effects.

A well-balanced diet that includes a variety of zinc-rich foods contributes to meeting your nutritional needs.

If you have specific concerns about zinc levels or dietary choices, consulting with a healthcare professional or a registered dietitian can provide personalized guidance.

Antioxidant-Rich Superfoods

Antioxidant-rich superfoods are nutrient-dense options that can help combat oxidative stress in the body, neutralizing harmful free radicals and contributing to overall health. Including a variety of these superfoods in your diet can provide numerous health benefits. Here are some antioxidant-rich superfoods:

- Berries: Blueberries, strawberries, raspberries, and blackberries are loaded with antioxidants, including anthocyanin's and vitamin C.

- Dark Leafy Greens: Kale, spinach, Swiss chard, and other dark leafy greens are rich in antioxidants like vitamins A, C, and E, as well as various phytochemicals.

- Nuts and Seeds: Almonds, walnuts, chia seeds, and flaxseeds are high in antioxidants, healthy fats, and fiber.

- Colorful Vegetables: Bell peppers, tomatoes, carrots, and sweet potatoes are packed with antioxidants such as beta-carotene, vitamin C, and lycopene.

- Fruits: In addition to berries, other fruits like apples, oranges, grapes, and kiwi provide a diverse range of antioxidants and essential vitamins.

- Green Tea: Green tea contains catechins, powerful antioxidants that have been associated with various health benefits, including improved heart health.

- Dark Chocolate: Dark chocolate with a high cocoa content is rich in flavonoids and antioxidants. Moderation is key due to its high calorie density.

- Turmeric: The active compound in turmeric, curcumin, has potent antioxidant and anti-inflammatory properties. It is commonly used in traditional cuisines and can be added to various dishes.

- Legumes: Beans, lentils, and chickpeas are excellent sources of antioxidants, fiber, and plant-based proteins.

- Fish: Fatty fish like salmon, mackerel, and trout are not only rich in omega-3 fatty acids but also contain selenium, a trace element with antioxidant properties.

- Seaweed: Edible seaweed, such as nori and wakame, is a source of antioxidants, vitamins, and minerals.

- Avocado: Avocado contains various antioxidants, including lutein, zeaxanthin, and vitamin E. It also provides healthy monounsaturated fats.

- Red Grapes: Red grapes, especially when consumed as red wine, contain resveratrol, a compound with antioxidant and anti-inflammatory properties.

- Broccoli: Broccoli and other cruciferous vegetables contain sulforaphane, a potent antioxidant with potential health benefits.

- Pomegranate: Pomegranate is rich in punicalagins and anthocyanins, contributing to its strong antioxidant properties.

Incorporating a variety of these antioxidant-rich superfoods into your diet can contribute to overall health and well-being. It's essential to maintain a balanced and diverse eating pattern to ensure you receive a broad spectrum of nutrients and antioxidants.

If you have specific dietary concerns or health conditions, consulting with a healthcare professional or a registered dietitian is advisable for personalized guidance.

Harnessing the Power of Berries

Berries, with their vibrant colors and delicious flavors, are not only a delightful addition to meals but also pack a powerful nutritional punch.

These small fruits are rich in a variety of antioxidants, vitamins, and minerals, offering numerous health benefits. Here's a closer look at how to harness the power of berries for your well-being:

- Abundance of Antioxidants: Berries, such as blueberries, strawberries, raspberries, and blackberries, are loaded with antioxidants. These compounds, including anthocyanin's, quercetin, and resveratrol, help combat oxidative stress, neutralizing harmful free radicals in the body.

- Heart Health: The antioxidants in berries contribute to cardiovascular health by reducing inflammation and improving blood vessel function. Regular consumption of berries has been associated with a lower risk of heart disease.

- Brain Boost: Berries have been linked to cognitive benefits, including improved memory and a slower rate of cognitive decline with age.
The antioxidants in berries may play a role in protecting brain cells and supporting overall brain health.

- Rich in Vitamins and Minerals: Berries are a good source of essential vitamins such as vitamin C, which supports immune function and skin health. They also provide minerals like potassium and manganese, contributing to overall nutritional well-being.

- Weight Management: Berries are relatively low in calories and high in fiber, making them a satisfying and nutritious snack. The fiber content helps promote feelings of fullness and supports digestive health.

- Diabetes Management: Some studies suggest that the antioxidants in berries may help improve insulin sensitivity and regulate blood sugar levels, making them a valuable addition to the diet for those managing diabetes.

- Anti-Inflammatory Properties: Chronic inflammation is linked to various health conditions, including heart disease and certain cancers. Berries' antioxidant and anti-inflammatory properties may contribute to reducing inflammation in the body.

- Skin Health: The vitamins and antioxidants in berries play a role in promoting skin health. They contribute to collagen production, helping maintain skin elasticity and a youthful appearance.

- Versatility in Culinary Use: Berries are incredibly versatile and can be easily incorporated into various dishes. Add them to smoothies, yogurt, salads, or enjoy them on their own as a refreshing snack.

- Seasonal Variety: Berries come in a variety of types and colors, and different berries may have unique nutritional profiles. Eating a mix of berries provides a broad spectrum of nutrients and flavors.

To harness the power of berries, aim to include a variety of these fruits in your daily diet. Whether fresh or frozen, berries offer a convenient and delicious way to boost your overall health. However, it's crucial to maintain a balanced diet that includes a variety of nutrient-rich foods for comprehensive nutrition.

If you have a particular dietary issues or health conditions, consider consulting your healthcare professional or a registered dietitian for personalized advice.

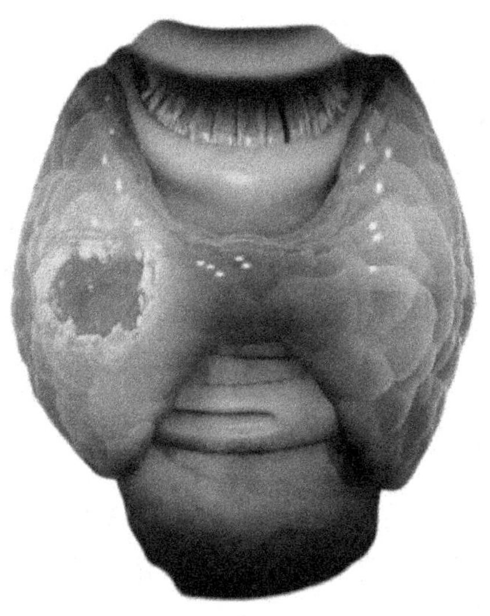

CHAPTER 4

Resetting Your Plate - Recipes for Thyroid Support

Maintaining a thyroid-friendly diet is crucial for supporting optimal thyroid function. By incorporating nutrient-dense and balanced meals into your routine, you can provide essential vitamins and minerals that contribute to thyroid health.

Here are a few recipes designed to support thyroid function:

1. Seaweed Salad with Salmon:

Ingredients:

- Seaweed (nori, wakame, or arame)
- Grilled salmon fillets
- Cucumber, julienned
- Carrot, shredded
- Sesame seeds
- Soy sauce
- Rice vinegar
- Sesame oil

Instructions:

- Soak seaweed according to package instructions.
- Mix seaweed with julienned cucumber, shredded carrot, and grilled salmon.
- In a separate bowl, whisk together soy sauce, rice vinegar, and sesame oil for the dressing.
- Toss the salad with the dressing, sprinkle sesame seeds, and serve.

2. Quinoa and Veggie Stir-Fry:

Ingredients:

- Quinoa, cooked
- Mixed vegetables (broccoli, bell peppers, carrots, and spinach)
- Tofu or lean chicken breast, cubed
- Garlic, minced
- Ginger, grated
- Soy sauce
- Olive oil

Instructions:

- In olive oil, sauté the ginger and garlic until aromatic.

- Add tofu or chicken and cook until browned.

- Stir in mixed vegetables and cook until tender-crisp.

- Add cooked quinoa and soy sauce, toss until well combined, and serve.

3. Berry and Spinach Smoothie:

Ingredients:

- Spinach leaves

- Mixed berries (blueberries, strawberries, raspberries)

- Greek yogurt

- Almond milk

- Chia seeds

Instructions:

- Blend spinach, mixed berries, Greek yogurt, and almond milk until smooth.

- Pour into a glass and sprinkle chia seeds on top for added nutrients.

4. Salmon and Avocado Wrap:

Ingredients:

- Grilled salmon flakes
- Whole-grain tortilla
- Avocado slices
- Spinach leaves
- Greek yogurt sauce (mix yogurt with lemon juice and dill)

Instructions:

- Lay out a tortilla and spread the Greek yogurt sauce.
- Layer with grilled salmon, avocado slices, and spinach leaves.
- Roll the tortilla and secure with toothpicks, if needed.

5. Roasted Vegetable Bowl:

Ingredients:

- Sweet potatoes, cubed
- Brussels sprouts, halved
- Red onion, sliced
- Chickpeas, drained and rinsed
- Olive oil

- Garlic powder, cumin, paprika

- Quinoa, cooked

Instructions:

- Toss sweet potatoes, Brussels sprouts, red onion, and chickpeas with olive oil and spices.

- Bake in the oven until cooked through and golden.

- Place on top of prepared quinoa for serving.

These recipes emphasize whole, nutrient-dense foods that provide essential nutrients for thyroid support. Remember to customize your diet based on individual preferences and dietary needs.

Additionally, consulting with a healthcare professional or a registered dietitian can offer personalized advice for maintaining a thyroid-friendly eating plan.

Breakfast Boosters for Thyroid Reset Diet: Fueling Your Day with Nutrient-Rich Morning Choices

For good reason, breakfast is frequently heralded as the most significant meal of the day. A well-balanced morning meal provides the energy and essential nutrients needed to kick start your metabolism and keep you alert and focused throughout the day.

Consider incorporating these breakfast boosters into your morning routine for a nutritious and satisfying start:

1. Oatmeal Power Bowl:

Ingredients:

- Rolled oats
- Almond milk or your preferred milk
- Chia seeds
- Fresh berries
- Sliced bananas
- Nuts and seeds (walnuts, flaxseeds, or almonds)
- Greek yogurt

Instructions:

- Cook oats with almond milk and chia seeds.
- Top with fresh berries, sliced bananas, a dollop of Greek yogurt, and a sprinkle of nuts and seeds.

2. Protein-Packed Smoothie:

Ingredients:

- Spinach or kale leaves
- Frozen mixed berries
- Greek yogurt
- Protein powder (optional)
- Almond milk or water

Instructions:

- Blend spinach, frozen berries, Greek yogurt, and protein powder with almond milk until smooth.
- Pour into a glass and enjoy a protein-packed, nutrient-rich smoothie.

3. Avocado Toast with Eggs:

Ingredients:

- Whole-grain bread
- Ripe avocado
- Poached or fried eggs
- Salt and pepper
- Optional toppings: cherry tomatoes, red pepper flakes, or feta cheese

Instructions:

- Mash ripe avocado and spread it on toasted whole-grain bread.
- Top with poached or fried eggs and season with salt and pepper.
- Customize with additional toppings for extra flavor and nutrients.

4. Yogurt Parfait:

Ingredients:

- Greek yogurt
- Granola (preferably low in added sugars)
- Fresh fruit (berries, kiwi, or mango)
- Honey or maple syrup (optional)

Instructions:

- Layer Greek yogurt with granola and fresh fruit in a glass or bowl.

- For sweetness, drizzle with maple syrup or honey.

5. Chia Seed Pudding:

Ingredients:

- Chia seeds
- Almond milk or coconut milk
- Vanilla extract
- Fresh fruit or berries
- Nuts or shredded coconut for topping

Instructions:

• Combine almond milk, vanilla essence, and chia seeds.

- Refrigerate overnight or for a few hours until it reaches a pudding-like consistency.
- Top with fresh fruit and nuts before serving.

6. Whole Grain Pancakes with Nut Butter:

Ingredients:

- Whole grain pancake mix
- Nut butter (almond, peanut, or cashew)
- Sliced bananas or berries

Instructions:

- Prepare whole grain pancakes according to package instructions.
- Spread a layer of nut butter on top and garnish with sliced bananas or berries.

Tips for Breakfast Success:

- Hydration: Rehydrate your body after a night of sleep by starting   your day with a glass of water.
- Balanced Plate: Include a mix of carbohydrates, protein, and healthy fats for sustained energy.
- Portion Control: Pay attention to portion proportions to prevent overindulging.
- Whole Foods: Opt for whole, minimally processed foods to maximize nutritional benefits.

By incorporating these breakfast boosters into your morning routine, you will not only enhance your nutrient intake but also set a positive tone for the day ahead. Customize these ideas to suit your taste preferences and dietary requirements, and consider consulting with a healthcare professional or a registered dietitian for personalized advice tailored to your individual needs.

Quinoa and Berry Breakfast Bowl

A Quinoa and Berry Breakfast Bowl is a nutritious and satisfying morning option that combines the protein-packed goodness of quinoa with the antioxidant-rich sweetness of berries.

This quick and easy breakfast provides a well-rounded mix of essential nutrients to kick start your day.

Ingredients:

- Cooked quinoa
- Mixed berries (blueberries, strawberries, raspberries)
- Greek yogurt
- Honey or maple syrup (optional)
- Nuts or seeds for crunch (almonds, chia seeds, or pumpkin seeds)

Instructions:

- Spoon a serving of cooked quinoa into a bowl.
- Top with a generous handful of mixed berries for natural sweetness and a burst of antioxidants.
- Add a dollop of Greek yogurt for protein and creaminess.

- Drizzle with honey or maple syrup if you prefer a touch of sweetness.
- Sprinkle with your choice of nuts or seeds for added texture and nutritional value.

Benefits:

- Protein: Quinoa is a complete protein source, offering all nine essential amino acids.
- Antioxidants: Antioxidants found in berries help the body fight oxidative stress.
- Fiber: Both quinoa and berries contribute to your daily fiber intake, supporting digestive health.
- Micronutrients: This breakfast bowl provides essential vitamins and minerals, promoting overall well-being.

Customization:

Feel free to personalize your Quinoa and Berry Breakfast Bowl by adding extras such as sliced bananas, a dash of cinnamon, or a sprinkle of coconut flakes. Adjust the sweetness to your liking and experiment with different berry combinations for variety.

This breakfast bowl is not only delicious but also a versatile and nutrient-dense way to start your day on a healthy note. Whether you're looking for a quick weekday breakfast or a leisurely weekend treat, the Quinoa and Berry Breakfast Bowl offers a delightful fusion of flavors and nutritional benefits.

Energizing Lunch Ideas for Thyroid Health

Supporting your thyroid health through a balanced and nutrient-dense lunch is essential. These energizing lunch ideas are crafted with ingredients that can contribute to thyroid function and overall well-being:

1. Salmon and Quinoa Salad:

Ingredients:

- Grilled or baked salmon
- Quinoa, cooked
- Mixed greens (spinach, arugula, kale)
- Cherry tomatoes
- Avocado slices
- Lemon-tahini dressing

Instructions:

- Combine grilled salmon, quinoa, mixed greens, cherry tomatoes, and avocado in a bowl.
- Drizzle with a lemon-tahini dressing for a flavorful and thyroid-friendly salad.

2. Sweet Potato and Chickpea Buddha Bowl:

Ingredients:

- Roasted sweet potatoes
- Roasted chickpeas
- Quinoa or brown rice
- Steamed broccoli
- Sliced cucumber
- Greek yogurt-tahini sauce

Instructions:

- Assemble a bowl with roasted sweet potatoes, chickpeas, quinoa or brown rice, steamed broccoli, and sliced cucumber.
- Drizzle with a Greek yogurt-tahini sauce for a nourishing and energizing lunch.

3. Turkey and Vegetable Stir-Fry:

Ingredients:

- Sliced turkey breast

- Stir-fry vegetables (bell peppers, broccoli, snap peas)

- Quinoa or cauliflower rice

- Ginger-garlic soy sauce

Instructions:

- Stir-fry sliced turkey with a variety of vegetables in a pan.

- Serve over quinoa or cauliflower rice, drizzled with a ginger-garlic soy sauce.

4. Spinach and Berry Salad with Chicken:

Ingredients:

- Grilled chicken breast

- Fresh spinach leaves

- Mixed berries (blueberries, strawberries)

- Walnuts or almonds

- Feta cheese

- Balsamic vinaigrette dressing

Instructions:

- Combine grilled chicken, fresh spinach, mixed berries, nuts, and feta cheese in a salad bowl.
- Dress with balsamic vinaigrette for a vibrant and thyroid-supportive salad.

5. Mango and Shrimp Quinoa Bowl:

Ingredients:

- Grilled shrimp
- Quinoa, cooked
- Mango cubes
- Red onion, finely chopped
- Cilantro
- Lime dressing

Instructions:

- Mix grilled shrimp, quinoa, mango cubes, red onion, and cilantro in a bowl.
- Drizzle with a lime dressing for a tropical-inspired and thyroid-friendly lunch.

6. Vegetarian Lentil Soup:

Ingredients:

- Green or brown lentils
- Carrots, celery, and onions
- Spinach or kale
- Vegetable broth
- Turmeric, cumin, and garlic for seasoning

Instructions:

- Cook lentils with diced vegetables, spinach or kale, vegetable broth, and seasonings.
- Enjoy a hearty and thyroid-supportive vegetarian lentil soup.

Tips for Thyroid-Friendly Lunches:

- Iodine-Rich Choices: Incorporate iodine-rich foods like seaweed, fish, and dairy to support thyroid function.
- Selenium Sources: Include selenium-rich foods like nuts, seeds, and lean meats to promote thyroid health.
- Whole Foods: Choose whole, minimally processed foods to maximize nutritional benefits.

- Hydration: Drink plenty of water throughout the day to stay hydrated.

These energizing lunch ideas are not only delicious but also designed to provide nutrients that can support thyroid health.

As always, it's essential to consider individual dietary needs and consult with a healthcare professional or a registered dietitian for personalized advice, especially if you have specific concerns about your thyroid health.

Nourishing Dinner Delights for Thyroid Reset

Dinner is an excellent opportunity to nourish your body and support thyroid health with nutrient-dense and balanced meals.

Here are some dinner ideas crafted with ingredients known for their potential benefits in promoting thyroid function:

1. Grilled Salmon with Roasted Vegetables:

Ingredients:

- Grilled salmon fillets
- Sweet potatoes, cubed
- Brussels sprouts, halved
- Olive oil, garlic, and rosemary for seasoning

Instructions:

- Season salmon fillets with herbs and grill until cooked.
- Roast sweet potatoes and Brussels sprouts with olive oil, garlic, and rosemary.
- Serve the grilled salmon over the bed of roasted vegetables for a thyroid-supportive dinner.

2. Turmeric Chickpea Stew:

Ingredients:

- Chickpeas, cooked
- Tomatoes, diced
- Spinach leaves
- Turmeric, cumin, and coriander for seasoning
- Quinoa or brown rice

Instructions:

- Cook chickpeas with diced tomatoes, spinach, and a blend of turmeric, cumin, and coriander.
- Serve over quinoa or brown rice for a nourishing and flavorful stew.

3. Chicken and Vegetable Stir-Fry:

Ingredients:

- Sliced chicken breast
- Mixed stir-fried veggies, such as carrots, broccoli, and bell peppers
- Quinoa or cauliflower rice
- Ginger and garlic for seasoning

Instructions:

- Stir-fry sliced chicken with a variety of vegetables, seasoned with ginger and garlic.
- Serve over quinoa or cauliflower rice for a thyroid-friendly stir-fry.

4. Mushroom and Spinach Quinoa Risotto:

Ingredients:

- Quinoa, cooked
- Mushrooms, sliced
- Spinach leaves
- Parmesan cheese
- Vegetable broth
- Garlic and thyme for flavor

Instructions:

- Sauté sliced mushrooms and garlic in a pan.
- Add cooked quinoa, spinach, and vegetable broth. Cook until creamy.
- Finish with Parmesan cheese and thyme for a comforting and thyroid-supportive risotto.

5. Shrimp and Asparagus Stir-Fry:

Ingredients:

- Shrimp, peeled and deveined
- Asparagus spears, chopped
- Brown rice
- Sesame oil, soy sauce, and ginger for flavor

Instructions:

- Stir-fry shrimp and asparagus with sesame oil, soy sauce, and ginger.
- Serve over brown rice for a quick and nutritious shrimp stir-fry.

6. Lentil and Vegetable Curry:

Ingredients:

- Green or brown lentils
- Mixed vegetables (zucchini, carrots, bell peppers)
- Coconut milk
- Curry spices (turmeric, cumin, coriander)
- Basmati rice

Instructions:

- Cook lentils with mixed vegetables, coconut milk, and curry spices until tender.
- Serve over basmati rice for a flavorful and thyroid-friendly lentil curry.

Tips for Thyroid-Supportive Dinners:

- Omega-3 Fatty Acids: Include fatty fish like salmon or chia seeds for their omega-3 content.

- Fiber-Rich Choices: Opt for whole grains, legumes, and vegetables to boost fiber intake.

- Iodine and Selenium: Incorporate iodine-rich foods like seaweed and selenium-rich sources like Brazil nuts.

- Hydration: Drink plenty of water to stay hydrated throughout the evening.

These nourishing dinner ideas are designed to support thyroid health while providing a variety of flavors and nutrients.

As always, individual dietary needs vary, and consulting with a healthcare professional or a registered dietitian can offer personalized guidance, especially if you have specific concerns about your thyroid health.

Seaweed-Wrapped Salmon Rolls for Thyroid Reset Diet

These delightful seaweed-wrapped salmon rolls are a fusion of flavors, combining the richness of salmon with the umami taste of seaweed.

Packed with nutrients such as omega-3 fatty acids and iodine, this dish not only offers a delicious dining experience but also provides potential benefits for thyroid health.

Ingredients:

- Fresh salmon fillets, thinly sliced
- Nori seaweed sheets
- Avocado, thinly sliced
- Cucumber, julienned
- Sesame seeds (black or white), for garnish
- Soy sauce or tamari, for dipping

Instructions:

Prepare Salmon Slices:

- Ensure the salmon fillets are thinly sliced for easy rolling.
- Season the salmon slices with a touch of salt and pepper.

Assemble Ingredients:

- Arrange a nori sheet on a spotless surface.
- Place a few slices of avocado, julienned cucumber, and thinly sliced salmon on the nori.

Rolling Technique:

- Start rolling the seaweed sheet from one end, using a bamboo sushi rolling mat if available.
- Apply a bit of water along the edge of the nori sheet to help seal the roll.

Slice into Rolls:

- Once rolled, use a sharp knife to slice the seaweed-wrapped roll into bite-sized pieces.

Garnish and Serve:

- For more taste and texture, sprinkle sesame seeds on top.

- Arrange the rolls on a serving platter.

Dipping Sauce:

- Serve with soy sauce or tamari on the side for dipping.

Tips for Seaweed-Wrapped Salmon Rolls:

- Fresh Ingredients: Use fresh and high-quality ingredients, especially when it comes to the salmon, to enhance the overall flavor.

- Experiment with Fillings: Feel free to customize the rolls with other ingredients like mango slices, radishes, or a thin layer of wasabi for added complexity.

- Iodine Boost: Seaweed is a rich source of iodine, which is essential for thyroid function. Including seaweed in your diet in moderation can contribute to iodine intake.

- Serving Suggestions: Accompany the rolls with pickled ginger and wasabi for a traditional sushi experience.

- Variation: If you prefer a grain-free option, you can replace the rice typically found in sushi rolls with cauliflower rice.

These seaweed-wrapped salmon roll not only make for a visually appealing dish but also offer a nutritious combination of omega-3s, iodine, and other essential nutrients.

As with any dietary considerations, it's advisable to consult with a healthcare professional or a registered dietitian, especially if you have specific concerns about your thyroid health or dietary needs. Enjoy these rolls as a flavorful and health-conscious addition to your culinary repertoire.

Snacks and Sides for Thyroid Reset Diet

Maintaining a thyroid-friendly diet involves incorporating nutrient-dense snacks and sides that provide essential vitamins and minerals. Here are some delicious options to keep you satisfied between meals and complement your thyroid reset journey:

Snacks:

Greek Yogurt Parfait:

Greek yogurt with a handful of mixed berries and a sprinkle of nuts or seeds. The yogurt provides probiotics, while berries offer antioxidants, and nuts or seeds add healthy fats.

Roasted Chickpeas:

Toss chickpeas with olive oil and seasonings like cumin and paprika, then roast until crispy. Chickpeas are a good source of protein and fiber.

Guacamole with Veggie Sticks:

Fresh guacamole paired with carrot and cucumber sticks. Avocados contribute healthy fats, and the veggies provide vitamins and minerals.

Seaweed Snacks:

Crispy seaweed snacks offer some low calorie option rich in iodine, an essential nutrient for thyroid function.

Nuts and Seeds Mix:

Create a trail mix with a variety of nuts and seeds, such as almonds, walnuts, sunflower seeds, and pumpkin seeds. These provide a mix of healthy fats, protein, and minerals.

Dark Chocolate and Almonds:

A small serving of dark chocolate paired with almonds. Dark chocolate contains antioxidants, while almonds provide protein and vitamin E.

Sides:

- **Quinoa Salad:** Quinoa mixed with diced vegetables, such as cucumber, cherry tomatoes, and bell peppers. Dress with olive oil, lemon juice, and herbs for a refreshing side dish.

- **Steamed Broccoli with Tahini:** Steam broccoli until tender and drizzle with a tahini dressing. Broccoli is rich in fiber, and tahini adds healthy fats.

- **Sweet Potato Wedges:** Roast sweet potato wedges with a sprinkle of cinnamon. A good source of beta-carotene, which is a precursor to vitamin A, is sweet potatoes.

- **Cauliflower Hummus:** Replace traditional chickpeas with cauliflower in hummus for a lower-carb option. Serve with veggie sticks for dipping.

- **Sautéed Spinach with Garlic:** Sauté spinach in olive oil with minced garlic for a quick and nutrient-packed side. Spinach is rich in iron and other vitamins.

- **Quinoa Stuffed Bell Peppers:** Mix quinoa with black beans, corn, and spices, then stuff bell peppers and bake until tender. Quinoa provides protein, and the peppers add color and vitamins.

Tips for Snacks and Sides on a Thyroid Reset Diet:

- **Balance Macronutrients:** Include a mix of carbohydrates, proteins, and healthy fats to keep energy levels stable.

- **Portion Control:** Be mindful of portion sizes to maintain overall caloric balance.

- **Incorporate Iodine-Rich Foods:** Seaweed, fish, and dairy can contribute to iodine intake, supporting thyroid function.

- **Hydration:** Stay well-hydrated by drinking water throughout the day.

- **Whole, Minimally Processed Foods:** Choose snacks and sides that are as close to their natural state as possible for maximum nutritional benefits.

These snacks and sides not only support thyroid health but also add variety and flavor to your diet. As with any dietary changes, it's recommended to consult with a healthcare professional or a registered dietitian, especially if you have specific concerns about your thyroid health or dietary needs.

Enjoy these snacks and sides as part of your balanced and thyroid-friendly eating plan.

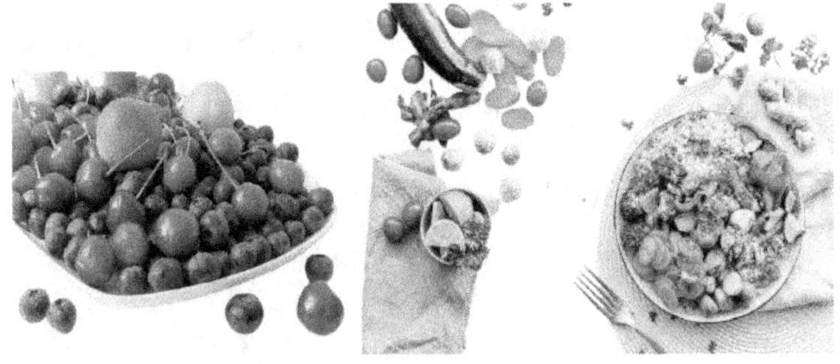

Thyroid-Friendly Smoothie for Resetting Your Diet

A well-crafted smoothie can be a delicious and nutritious addition to a thyroid reset diet. Packed with ingredients that support thyroid health, this smoothie combines flavors for a refreshing and nourishing drink.

Ingredients:

- **Spinach or Kale:** Rich in vitamins A and K, as well as iron. These leafy greens add a nutritional boost without overpowering the flavor.

- **Berries (Blueberries, Strawberries):** Loaded with antioxidants, particularly anthocyanins, which may help combat oxidative stress.

- **Greek Yogurt:** A good source of protein and probiotics, contributing to gut health.

- **Chia Seeds or Flaxseeds:** Provide omega-3 fatty acids, fiber, and additional nutrients for overall well-being.

- **Coconut Water or Almond Milk:** Hydrating and adds a smooth texture to the smoothie. Almond milk also contributes vitamin E.

- **Banana:** Adds natural sweetness and a source of potassium.

- **Brazil Nuts:** Rich in selenium, a trace element essential for thyroid function.

- **Iodine-Rich Foods (optional):** Consider adding a small amount of iodine-rich ingredients like seaweed or iodized salt.

Instructions:

Prepare Ingredients:

- Wash and measure the desired amount of spinach or kale.

- Rinse berries and slice the banana.

- Measure the desired amount of Greek yogurt and coconut water or almond milk.

- If using chia seeds or flaxseeds, measure accordingly.

- Blend: In a blender, combine all the ingredients.

- Blend until smooth, adjusting the liquid to achieve your preferred consistency.

Optional Additions:

- For additional flavor and nutrition, consider adding a teaspoon of honey, a dash of cinnamon, or a scoop of protein powder.
- Serve and Enjoy: Pour the smoothie into a glass and savor the thyroid-friendly goodness.

Tips for a Thyroid-Friendly Smoothie:

- **Balance Macros**: Ensure a balance of carbohydrates, protein, and healthy fats for sustained energy.

- **Incorporate Iodine-Rich Ingredients**: If you're using seaweed or iodized salt, be mindful of the quantity to meet but not exceed recommended iodine intake.

- **Limit Added Sugars:** Opt for natural sweetness from fruits rather than excessive added sugars.

- **Variety is Key:** Experiment with different greens, fruits, and seeds to diversify your nutrient intake.

- **Hydrate:** Coconut water provides hydration, and staying well-hydrated is essential for overall health.

- **Consult with a Professional:** If you have specific concerns about your thyroid health, consult with a healthcare professional or a registered dietitian for personalized advice.

This thyroid-friendly smoothie is not only a tasty treat but also a convenient way to incorporate essential nutrients into your diet.

As with any dietary changes, individual needs vary, and it's advisable to seek professional advice to tailor your diet to your specific health requirements. Enjoy this smoothie as part of a well-rounded and thyroid-supportive eating plan.

CHAPTER 5

Crafting Thyroid-Supportive Meal Plans

Creating a thyroid-supportive meal plan involves incorporating nutrient-dense foods that provide essential vitamins and minerals known to support thyroid function. Here's a guide to help you craft a well-balanced and thyroid-friendly meal plan:

Key Components:

Iodine-Rich Foods: Include sources of iodine such as seaweed, fish, dairy, and iodized salt. Iodine is a crucial element for thyroid hormone synthesis.

Selenium Sources: Integrate selenium-rich foods like Brazil nuts, sunflower seeds, lean meats, and seafood. Selenium supports the conversion of thyroid hormones.

Omega-3 Fatty Acids: Choose fatty fish such as salmon, mackerel, or chia seeds and flaxseeds. Omega-3s are beneficial for reducing inflammation and supporting thyroid function.

Fruits and Vegetables: Opt for a variety of colorful fruits and vegetables, providing essential vitamins, minerals, and antioxidants. These contribute to overall well-being.

Protein-Rich Foods: Include lean protein sources like poultry, fish, beans, lentils, and tofu. Protein is crucial for thyroid hormone synthesis and transportation.

Whole Grains: Choose whole grains like quinoa, brown rice, and oats. Whole grains provide fiber, supporting digestive health and stabilizing blood sugar levels.

Healthy Fats: Include foods like avocados, almonds, seeds, and olive oil that are good sources of fat. The synthesis of hormones and the absorption of fat-soluble vitamins are both influenced by fats. Limit Processed Foods and Added Sugars, minimize processed foods and refined sugars, as they may contribute to inflammation and disrupt hormonal balance.

Weekly Meal Planning Guide:

Meal planning is a powerful tool that can help you achieve your nutritional goals, save time, and reduce stress around meals. Here's a comprehensive guide to creating a weekly meal plan:

1. Assess Your Goals and Preferences: Identify your nutritional goals, whether it's weight management, improving energy levels, or supporting specific health concerns.

Consider any dietary preferences, restrictions, or allergies.

2. Create a Weekly Calendar: Use a calendar or meal planning template to visualize your week.

Designate specific days for breakfast, lunch, dinner, and snacks.

3. Inventory and Shopping List: Take inventory of your pantry, fridge, and freezer to see what ingredients you already have.

Create a shopping list based on the ingredients needed for your planned meals.

4. Include Varieties of Foods: Every meal should aim to have a balance of the three macronutrients: fats, proteins, and carbohydrates.

Include a variety of fruits, vegetables, whole grains, lean proteins, and healthy fats.

5. Consider Batch Cooking: Plan meals that can be prepared in batches to save time during the week.

Cook grains, proteins, or sauces in larger quantities to use in multiple meals.

6. Theme Nights: Assign themes to certain nights to simplify planning (e.g., Meatless Monday, Taco Tuesday, Stir-Fry Wednesday).

7. Flexibility for Leftovers: Plan for leftovers to minimize food waste and simplify meal preparation.

Designate a specific day to eat leftovers or get creative with repurposing them.

8. Mindful Portion Control: Consider portion sizes to avoid overeating.

To promote portion management, use smaller bowls and plates.

9. Hydration: Plan for hydration by incorporating water, herbal teas, or infused water throughout the day.

Limit sugary drinks and excessive caffeine.

10. Snacks: Include healthy snacks to curb hunger between meals.

Select snacks that provide you with continuous energy by combining fiber, protein, and healthy fats.

11. Meal Prep: Dedicate a specific time for meal prep each week.

Wash, chop, and prepare ingredients in advance for easy assembly during busy days.

Sample Weekly Meal Plan:

Monday:

Breakfast: Greek yogurt parfait with berries and nuts

Lunch: Quinoa and vegetable stir-fry with tofu

Dinner: Baked salmon, sweet potato wedges, and steamed broccoli

Tuesday:

Breakfast: Smoothie with spinach, banana, chia seeds, and almond milk

Lunch: Chickpea salad with mixed greens, tomatoes, cucumber, and feta

Dinner: Turkey and vegetable chili with a side of brown rice

Wednesday:

Breakfast: Oatmeal with sliced apples, cinnamon, and a dollop of almond butter

Lunch: salad with avocado, shrimp, and mixed greens

Dinner: Vegetarian lentil soup with whole-grain bread

Thursday:

Breakfast: Poached eggs and mashed avocado on whole grain bread

Lunch: Quinoa stuffed bell peppers with a side of Greek yogurt

Dinner: Grilled chicken breast, quinoa, and roasted Brussels sprouts

Friday:

Breakfast: Chia seed pudding with coconut milk and mixed berries

Lunch: Mediterranean chickpea bowl with couscous and tzatziki

Dinner: Tofu stir-fried with brown rice and broccoli

Tips for Success:

- Be Realistic: Consider your schedule and choose meals that align with the time you have available for preparation.

- Rotate Favorites: Include favorite meals regularly to maintain enjoyment and adherence to the plan.

- Stay Flexible: Allow for flexibility and be open to adjusting the plan based on unexpected events or changing preferences.

- Variety is Key: Embrace variety to ensure a broad spectrum of nutrients and prevent culinary boredom.

- Observe your Body: Observe your body's signals of hunger and fullness. As necessary, adjust the portion sizes.

- Review and Reflect: At the end of the week, reflect on what worked well and what could be improved. Use this feedback for future meal planning.

Remember that meal planning is a dynamic process that can be adapted to suit your needs and lifestyle. Experiment with different recipes, flavors, and cuisines to keep your meals exciting and enjoyable.

As always, consider consulting with a registered dietitian or healthcare professional for personalized guidance based on your specific health goals and dietary requirements.

Smart Substitutions and Ingredient Swaps for Thyroid Reset Diet:

Making thoughtful ingredient choices and substitutions is a key aspect of crafting a thyroid-friendly diet. Here are smart swaps and substitutions to consider for a thyroid reset diet:

1. Replace Refined Grains with Whole Grains: Swap white rice for quinoa, brown rice, or farro to increase fiber and nutrient content.

2. Choose Lean Proteins: Opt for lean protein sources like chicken, turkey, tofu, or legumes instead of processed or fatty meats.

3. Use Healthy Fats: Substitute saturated fats with healthier options such as avocados, nuts, seeds, and olive oil.

4. Low-Fat Dairy Alternatives: Choose low-fat or fat-free dairy options like skim milk or Greek yogurt instead of full-fat alternatives.

5. Go for Low-Glycemic Sweeteners: Use natural sweeteners with a lower glycemic index, such as honey, maple syrup, or stevia, instead of refined sugars.

6. Include Iodine-Rich Alternatives: Incorporate iodine-rich foods like seaweed or sea vegetables instead of relying solely on iodized salt.

7. Prefer Omega-3 Rich Choices: Choose fatty fish like salmon or mackerel over less omega-3-rich options to support thyroid health.

8. Limit Processed Foods: Minimize processed foods that often contain hidden sugars, unhealthy fats, and additives.

9. Swap Regular Salt for Sea Salt: Consider using sea salt instead of regular table salt for a potential boost in trace minerals.

10. Use Coconut Oil in Moderation: While coconut oil can be a healthy choice, use it in moderation due to its high saturated fat content.

11. Opt for Non-Dairy Milk Alternatives: Choose non-dairy milk options like almond, soy, or coconut milk instead of cow's milk if you have lactose sensitivity.

12. Experiment with Gluten-Free Grains: If sensitive to gluten, try gluten-free grains like quinoa, buckwheat, or rice instead of wheat-based products.

13. Choose Organic Produce: When possible, opt for organic fruits and vegetables to reduce exposure to pesticides and support overall health.

14. Herbs and Spices Instead of Excess Salt: Flavor dishes with herbs, spices, and seasonings to reduce reliance on excessive salt for taste.

15. Minimize Caffeine and Alcohol: Limit caffeine and alcohol intake, choosing herbal teas or water with lemon as alternative beverages.

16. Explore Plant-Based Proteins: Integrate plant-based proteins such as beans, lentils, and tofu as alternatives to animal products.

17. Select Low-Sugar Snacks: Choose snacks with lower sugar content, like fresh fruit, nuts, or vegetable sticks with hummus.

18. Mindful Cooking Methods: Opt for cooking methods like baking, grilling, steaming, or sautéing instead of deep-frying to preserve nutritional content.

19. Avoid Artificial Additives: Read labels and avoid foods with artificial colors, flavors, and preservatives.

20. Stay Hydrated with Water: Prioritize water as the main beverage to stay adequately hydrated.

Tips for Success:

- Gradual Changes: Implement changes gradually to allow your taste buds and habits to adjust.
- Observe Your Body: Observe your body's reaction to various components and make necessary adjustments.
- Personalize Your Approach: Everyone's body reacts differently, so personalize your diet based on your specific needs and preferences.

- Consult with Professionals: If you have specific concerns or health conditions, consult with a healthcare professional or a registered dietitian for personalized advice.

Making smart substitutions and mindful ingredient choices can contribute to a thyroid-friendly diet that supports overall well-being.

As with any dietary changes, it's essential to consider individual needs and consult with a healthcare professional or a registered dietitian for personalized guidance.

Elevating Flavors with Herbs and Spices for Thyroid Reset Diet:

Enhancing the taste of thyroid-friendly meals doesn't have to rely on excessive salt or processed condiments. Instead, you can elevate flavors by incorporating a variety of herbs and spices, not only to make your dishes delicious but also to provide potential health benefits. Here's a guide on how to use herbs and spices to add depth and richness to your thyroid reset diet:

1. Turmeric:

Flavor Profile: Warm and slightly bitter.

Health Benefits: Contains curcumin, known for its anti-inflammatory properties.

Use in: Curries, soups, roasted vegetables, and rice dishes.

2. Ginger:

Flavor Profile: Spicy, warm, and slightly sweet.

Health Benefits: Anti-inflammatory and aids digestion.

Use in: Stir-fries, smoothies, tea, and marinades.

3. Rosemary:

Flavor Profile: Woody and aromatic.

Health Benefits: Rich in antioxidants and may support digestion.

Use in: Roasted meats, potatoes, bread, and soups.

4. Cinnamon:

Flavor Profile: Sweet and warm.

Health Benefits: might aid in controlling blood sugar levels.

Use in: Oatmeal, smoothies, baked goods, and curries.

5. Garlic:

Flavor Profile: Pungent and savory.

Health Benefits: Contains allicin, known for its antibacterial properties.

Use in: Sauces, roasted vegetables, soups, and marinades.

6. Basil:

Flavor Profile: Sweet and slightly peppery.

Health Benefits: Rich in antioxidants.

Use in: Pasta dishes, salads, soups, and sauces.

7. Cumin:

Flavor Profile: Earthy and warm.

Health Benefits: May aid digestion and provide iron.

Use in: Curries, chili, roasted vegetables, and rice dishes.

8. Parsley:

Flavor Profile: Fresh and slightly peppery.

Health Benefits: Contains vitamins A and C.

Use in: Salads, soups, marinades, and as a garnish.

9. Thyme:

Flavor Profile: Earthy and slightly floral.

Health Benefits: Contains antioxidants and may have antimicrobial properties.

Use in: Roasted meats, soups, stews, and vegetables.

Tips for Incorporating Herbs and Spices:

- Experiment Boldly: Don't be afraid to try new combinations and experiment with bold flavors.
- Fresh vs. Dried: Both fresh and dried herbs have their place. Use fresh herbs for a vibrant taste and dried herbs for convenience.
- Layer Flavors: Build layers of flavor by adding herbs and spices at different stages of cooking.
- Balance is Key: Aim for a balanced mix of herbs and spices to create a harmonious taste.
- Consider Culinary Cultures: Explore herbs and spices commonly used in different cuisines for diverse flavor profiles.

- Garnishing: Use fresh herbs as a finishing touch to add brightness and freshness to a dish.
- Customize to Your Taste: Adjust the quantities of herbs and spices based on personal preference.

By embracing the diverse world of herbs and spices, you not only enhance the flavor of your meals but also introduce a variety of nutrients and potential health benefits to your thyroid reset diet.

Enjoy the culinary journey as you discover the wonderful tastes and aromas these natural flavor enhancers can bring to your dishes.

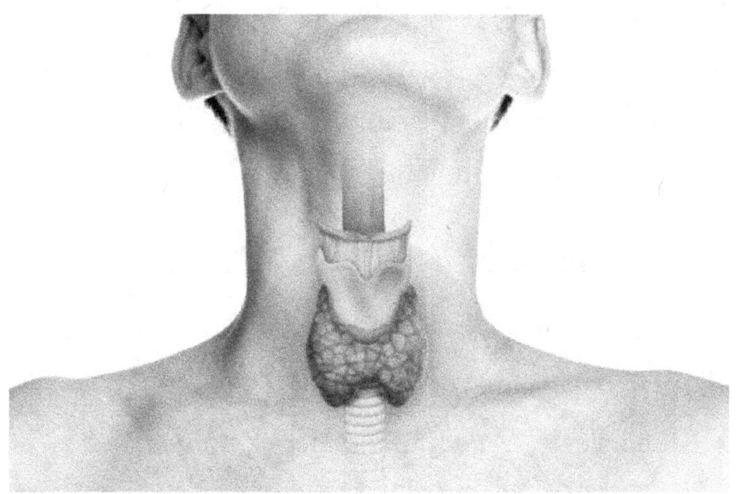

CHAPTER 6

Beyond the Plate - Lifestyle Tips for Thyroid Health

Maintaining a healthy thyroid goes beyond dietary choices; lifestyle factors also play a crucial role. Consider incorporating the following tips into your daily routine to support overall thyroid health:

Exercise Strategies for Thyroid Function

Regular physical activity is a vital component of a healthy lifestyle, and it can positively impact thyroid function. Incorporating exercise strategies that align with thyroid health can contribute to overall well-being. Here are some exercise tips to support thyroid function:

1. Cardiovascular Exercise:

- Type: Engage in aerobic exercises like walking, jogging, cycling, or swimming.
- Frequency: Aim for at least 150 minutes of moderate-intensity aerobic exercise per week.

- Benefits: Cardiovascular exercise supports metabolism and helps manage stress, both of which are beneficial for thyroid health.

2. Strength Training:

- Type: Include resistance training or strength training exercises.
- Frequency: At least twice a week, engage in strength training that focuses on your primary muscle groups.
- Benefits: Building lean muscle mass can boost metabolism and support overall energy expenditure.

3. Interval Training:

- Type: Incorporate high-intensity interval training (HIIT) workouts.
- Frequency: Include HIIT sessions 1-2 times per week.
- Benefits: HIIT can be efficient in burning calories and improving cardiovascular health, supporting thyroid function.

4. Yoga and Stretching:

- Type: Integrate yoga or stretching exercises.

- Frequency: Include yoga or stretching sessions regularly, especially focusing on poses that support the thyroid gland.
- Benefits: Yoga helps manage stress, improves flexibility, and may positively influence thyroid function.

5. Outdoor Activities:

- Type: Take advantage of outdoor activities like hiking, cycling, or jogging.
- Frequency: Enjoy outdoor exercises regularly for a change of scenery and exposure to natural sunlight, which supports vitamin D production.

6. Mind-Body Practices:

- Type: Incorporate mind-body practices like tai chi or qigong.
- Frequency: Engage in mind-body exercises regularly to promote relaxation and reduce stress.

7. Consistency is Key:

- Type: Choose exercises you enjoy and can sustain over the long term.

- Frequency: Consistency is more important than intensity. To maintain motivation, engage in things you enjoy.

8. Listen to Your Body:

- Type: Be mindful of your body's signals and adjust exercise intensity accordingly.
- Frequency: Rest when needed and allow for recovery days to prevent overtraining.

9. Warm-Up and Cool Down:

- Type: Always include warm-up and cool-down exercises.
- Frequency: Prioritize injury prevention by preparing your body before intense workouts and aiding recovery afterward.

Exercise is a valuable tool for supporting thyroid function, but it's important to tailor your workout routine to your individual needs and preferences.

Always consult with a healthcare professional or fitness expert, especially if you have underlying health conditions or concerns about thyroid health.

By incorporating a well-rounded and consistent exercise routine, you can contribute to overall thyroid health and enhance your overall well-being.

The Role of Yoga and Meditation for Thyroid Reset

Yoga and meditation can be powerful tools in promoting overall well-being, and specifically, they can play a supportive role in resetting and maintaining thyroid health. Here's a look at the benefits of incorporating yoga and meditation into your routine for a thyroid reset:

1. Stress Reduction:

Yoga: Practices such as gentle yoga poses, restorative yoga, and yin yoga can help release physical tension and reduce stress.

Meditation: Mindful meditation techniques, such as deep breathing or guided imagery, can activate the body's relaxation response, alleviating stress.

2. Balancing Hormones:

Yoga: Certain yoga poses, like shoulder stands and fish pose, are believed to stimulate the thyroid gland, potentially helping to balance hormone levels.

Meditation: Mindful practices can influence the endocrine system, helping to regulate hormone production and balance.

3. Improved Sleep Quality:

Yoga: A regular yoga practice has been linked to improved sleep patterns, helping to regulate the circadian rhythm and promote restful sleep.

Meditation: Mindfulness meditation can calm the mind, making it easier to unwind and achieve better sleep.

4. Enhanced Circulation:

Yoga: Dynamic yoga styles, like vinyasa or power yoga, can enhance blood circulation, ensuring optimal delivery of nutrients to the thyroid gland.

Meditation: Practices that involve mindful breathing can improve overall circulation and oxygenation of the body.

5. Mind-Body Connection:

Yoga: Yoga emphasizes the mind-body connection, fostering awareness of physical sensations and promoting a sense of balance.

Meditation: Mindfulness meditation enhances the connection between the mind and body, helping to create a sense of harmony.

6. Reduced Inflammation:

Yoga: Regular yoga practice may contribute to reducing inflammation in the body, which is beneficial for thyroid health.

Meditation: Mindful practices have been associated with lower levels of inflammatory markers in the body.

7. Energy Regulation:

Yoga: Dynamic yoga practices can boost energy levels, helping to combat fatigue often associated with thyroid issues.

Meditation: Mindful meditation can increase alertness and mental clarity, contributing to sustained energy throughout the day.

8. Mindful Eating:

Yoga: The practice of mindful eating can be incorporated into yoga philosophy, promoting awareness of food choices and eating habits.

Meditation: Mindful meditation can enhance the awareness of hunger and fullness cues, supporting a balanced approach to nutrition.

9. Improved Mental Health:

Yoga: The combination of physical movement and breath awareness in yoga can positively impact mental health, reducing symptoms of anxiety and depression.

Meditation: Mindfulness meditation is recognized for its mental health benefits, providing a tool for stress management and emotional well-being.

10. Holistic Approach:

Yoga: Yoga, with its emphasis on holistic well-being, addresses physical, mental, and emotional aspects of health.

Meditation: Meditation complements the holistic approach, fostering a sense of inner calm and balance.

Incorporating Yoga and Meditation:

Start Slow: If new to yoga or meditation, begin with gentle practices and gradually increase intensity.

Consistency Matters: Regularity in practice is key to experiencing the full benefits. Aim for a balanced routine throughout the week.

Listen to Your Body: Pay attention to how your body responds to different practices and adjust accordingly.

Guidance from Professionals: Consider joining classes or seeking guidance from experienced instructors to ensure proper technique and progression.

Yoga and meditation offer a holistic approach to thyroid health, addressing both physical and mental aspects. While these practices can be supportive, it's crucial to work in collaboration with healthcare professionals to create a comprehensive plan that considers individual health needs.

Whether you're a beginner or experienced practitioner, integrating yoga and meditation into your routine can contribute positively to your overall well-being and thyroid health.

Stress Management Techniques for Thyroid Reset

Chronic stress can adversely impact thyroid function, making stress management a crucial component of a thyroid reset plan. Here are effective stress management techniques to incorporate into your routine for thyroid health:

1. Mindfulness Meditation:

Technique: Practice mindfulness meditation by focusing on your breath, observing thoughts without attachment, and being present in the moment.

Benefits: Reduces stress hormones, promotes relaxation, and enhances overall mental well-being.

2. Deep Breathing Exercises:

Technique: Engage in deep, diaphragmatic breathing. Inhale slowly through your nose, expanding your abdomen, hold briefly, and exhale slowly through your mouth.

Benefits: Activates the parasympathetic nervous system, inducing a calming effect and reducing stress.

3. Progressive Muscle Relaxation (PMR):

Technique: Systematically tense and then release different muscle groups, starting from your toes and working up to your head.

Benefits: Relieves physical tension, promotes relaxation, and reduces stress-related symptoms.

4. Guided Imagery and Visualization:

Technique: Close your eyes and visualize a peaceful scene or engage in guided imagery exercises to create a mental sanctuary.

Benefits: Shifts focus away from stressors, promoting relaxation and mental calmness.

5. Yoga and Tai Chi:

Technique: Engage in yoga poses or tai chi movements, incorporating breath awareness for a mind-body connection.

Benefits: Combines physical activity with mindfulness, promoting relaxation and stress relief.

6. Aromatherapy:

Technique: Use essential oils like lavender, chamomile, or bergamot through diffusers or diluted for massage.

Benefits: Aromas can have a calming effect, reducing stress and promoting a sense of well-being.

7. Journaling:

Technique: Write down your thoughts, feelings, and stressors in a journal.

Benefits: Provides an outlet for expressing emotions, gaining clarity, and reducing the mental burden of stress.

8. Nature Walks:

Technique: Spend time outdoors, taking leisurely walks in natural settings.

Benefits: Exposure to nature has been shown to lower stress levels and enhance mood.

9. Social Connections:

Technique: Maintain and nurture positive social connections with friends and family.

Benefits: Social support can act as a buffer against stress and contribute to overall well-being.

Effective stress management is integral to a thyroid reset plan. By incorporating these techniques into your daily life, you can create a resilient foundation for both your mental well-being and thyroid health. As stress is a personalized experience, it may be beneficial to experiment with various strategies to determine what resonates most with you. If stress persists or becomes overwhelming, consider seeking guidance from healthcare professionals for personalized support.

Prioritizing Quality Sleep for Thyroid Support

Quality sleep is foundational to overall health and plays a significant role in supporting optimal thyroid function. Here's why prioritizing quality sleep is crucial for thyroid health and practical tips to enhance your sleep routine:

Why Quality Sleep Matters for Thyroid Health

- Hormonal Regulation: Adequate sleep is essential for the proper regulation of hormones, including those involved in thyroid function. Sleep deprivation can disrupt the delicate balance of hormones, impacting thyroid health.

- Tissue Repair and Restoration: During sleep, the body undergoes crucial repair and restoration processes. Quality sleep supports tissue repair, cellular regeneration, and the overall maintenance of bodily functions, including those related to the thyroid.

- Circadian Rhythm Influence: The circadian rhythm, the body's internal clock, plays a role in regulating thyroid hormones. Disruptions in sleep patterns can affect this rhythm, potentially impacting thyroid function.

- Immune System Support: Quality sleep is linked to a robust immune system.
A well-functioning immune system contributes to overall health, preventing potential stressors that may impact the thyroid.

- Inflammation Reduction: Chronic sleep deprivation is associated with increased inflammation. Inflammation can negatively affect thyroid function and exacerbate existing thyroid conditions.

Tips for Prioritizing Quality Sleep:

- Consistent Sleep Schedule: Every day, including on weekends, go to bed and wake up at the same hour. The body's innate circadian rhythm is strengthened by consistency.

- Create a Relaxing Bedtime Routine: Develop a calming routine before bed, such as reading, gentle stretching, or practicing relaxation techniques. Avoid stimulating activities close to bedtime.

- Optimize Sleep Environment: Ensure your bedroom is conducive to sleep by maintaining a comfortable temperature, minimizing noise and light, and investing in a comfortable mattress and pillows.

- Limit Screen Time Before Bed: At least one hour before going to bed, limit your time spent using electronic devices with screens. The melatonin hormone, which promotes sleep, may be inhibited by the blue light that screens emit.

- Mindful Eating in the Evening: Avoid heavy meals close to bedtime. If you're hungry, choose a healthy, light snack. Limit caffeine and alcohol intake in the hours leading up to sleep.

- Stay Active During the Day: Regular exercise helps you sleep better. Every day, try to get in at least 30 minutes of moderate activity; however, stay away from intense workouts right before bed.

- Manage Stress: Incorporate stress management techniques, such as meditation, deep breathing exercises, or progressive muscle relaxation, into your evening routine to unwind before bed.

- Limit Naps: While short naps can be rejuvenating, avoid lengthy or late-afternoon naps that may interfere with nighttime sleep.

- Mind-Body Practices: Engage in mind-body practices like yoga or tai chi. These activities can promote relaxation and contribute to a more peaceful sleep.

- Evaluate Your Sleep Environment: Invest in a comfortable mattress and pillows, and ensure your bedroom is free from disruptions like excess light and noise.

- Seek Professional Guidance: If sleep difficulties persist, consult with a healthcare professional or sleep specialist for personalized advice and potential evaluation for sleep disorders.

- Consistency and Patience: Improving sleep habits takes time and consistency. It's essential to be patient as you implement changes to your sleep routine. If sleep problems persist, consult with a healthcare professional to identify underlying issues and receive personalized guidance.

Prioritizing quality sleep is a fundamental aspect of supporting thyroid health. By incorporating these tips into your routine and creating a conducive sleep environment, you can contribute to better overall well-being and optimize the conditions for a healthy thyroid function. Remember that individual sleep needs vary, so paying attention to your body's signals and making adjustments accordingly is key.

Conclusion

Nurturing Your Thyroid Journey

In conclusion, embarking on a thyroid reset journey through a carefully curated diet is a transformative and empowering endeavor. The recipes and insights within this cookbook aim to not only nourish your body but also to foster a harmonious relationship with your thyroid. As we celebrate the culmination of these pages, let it be a reminder that a thyroid-friendly diet is not merely a prescription; it is a celebration of flavors, a symphony of nutrients, and a conscious choice for your well-being.

This cookbook serves as a compass, guiding you through a culinary adventure where each ingredient is a note in the melody of thyroid support.

From iodine-rich foods to selenium-packed options, antioxidant-rich superfoods to zinc-packed delights, every recipe is crafted with intention to recalibrate, rejuvenate, and revitalize. We've explored the vitality of herbs and spices, harnessed the power of berries, and delved into the art of crafting meals that resonate with your thyroid's well-being.

As you reset your plate, remember that this journey is more than a collection of recipes; it is a holistic approach to embracing a lifestyle that nurtures your body and soul. Beyond the plate, the significance of exercise, stress management, and quality sleep have been highlighted — each playing a pivotal role in your thyroid reset.

May this cookbook not only be a source of delicious meals but also a guide to a mindful, thyroid-supportive lifestyle. Let it inspire you to listen to your body, savor the journey of crafting nourishing meals, and revel in the joy of prioritizing your health.

As you savor each bite, remember that you are taking a step towards a healthier, more vibrant version of yourself.

In the spirit of well-being, let this cookbook be a companion on your thyroid reset voyage, guiding you towards a path where your plate reflects the love and care you have for yourself.

Here's to a future filled with vitality, balance, and the countless joys that a thyroid-friendly lifestyle can bring. Happy cooking, happy healing, and cheers to a life well-nourished!

APPENDIX A: THYROID-FRIENDLY INGREDIENT LIST

This comprehensive list serves as a valuable resource for selecting ingredients that align with a thyroid-friendly diet. Incorporating these nutrient-rich foods into your meals can contribute to optimal thyroid function and overall well-being.

1. Iodine-Rich Foods:

- Seaweed (kelp, nori, wakame)
- Fish (cod, tuna, shrimp)
- Dairy products (yogurt, milk)
- Eggs
- Iodized salt (in moderation)

2. Selenium Sources:

- Brazil nuts
- Sunflower seeds
- Fish (tuna, halibut, sardines)
- Turkey

* Beef

3. Zinc-Packed Options:

* Pumpkin seeds
* Chickpeas
* Spinach
* Beef
* Lentils

4. Antioxidant-Rich Superfoods:

* Berries (blueberries, strawberries, raspberries)
* Dark leafy greens (kale, spinach)
* Nuts (walnuts, almonds)
* Tomatoes
* Green tea

5. Herbs and Spices for Flavor Enhancement:

* Turmeric
* Ginger
* Rosemary
* Cinnamon
* Garlic

6. Berries for Harnessing Power:

- Acai berries
- Goji berries
- Elderberries
- Cranberries
- Blackberries

7. Essential Nutrients for Thyroid Health:

- Omega-3 fatty acids (fatty fish, flaxseeds, chia seeds)
- Vitamins A and D (sweet potatoes, carrots, salmon)
- B-vitamins (whole grains, legumes, nuts)
- Iron (lean meats, beans, tofu)

8. Thyroid-Supportive Proteins:

- Lean poultry (chicken, turkey)
- Fatty fish (salmon, trout)
- Plant-based proteins (tofu, tempeh, lentils)
- Greek yogurt
- Eggs
- 9. Whole Grains and Fiber:
- Quinoa

- Brown rice

- Oats

- Whole wheat

- Barley

10. Fruits and Vegetables for Micronutrients:

- Leafy greens (spinach, kale)

- Cruciferous vegetables (broccoli, Brussels sprouts)

- Citrus fruits (oranges, grapefruits)

- Bell peppers

- Avocado

11. Dairy and Alternatives:

- Greek yogurt

- Milk (cow's milk, almond milk, soy milk)

- Cheese (in moderation)

- Cottage cheese

- Kefir

12. Hydration Choices:

- Water (plain or infused with herbs)

- Herbal teas (chamomile, peppermint)

- Coconut water

- Green tea (moderate caffeine)

13. Healthy Fats:

- Olive oil

- Avocado

- Nuts and seeds

- Fatty fish (salmon, mackerel)

14. Sweeteners and Alternatives:

- Honey (in moderation)

- Maple syrup

- Stevia

- Coconut sugar

Use this appendix as a guide when planning your meals, ensuring that your choices align with the principles of a thyroid-friendly diet. Remember to consult with healthcare professionals for personalized advice based on individual health needs.

APPENDIX B: QUICK REFERENCE COOKING TIPS

Enhance your culinary experience with these quick and handy cooking tips. Whether you're a seasoned chef or just starting your kitchen adventures, these suggestions will elevate your thyroid-friendly cooking:

1. Flavorful Herbs and Spices:

Tip: Experiment with thyroid-friendly herbs like turmeric, ginger, and rosemary to add depth and flavor to your dishes.

2. Iodine Awareness:

Tip: While iodine is essential, moderation is key. Be mindful of iodized salt and seafood intake to maintain a balanced iodine level.

3. Omega-3 Boost:

Tip: Include omega-3-rich ingredients like fatty fish, flaxseeds, and chia seeds for their anti-inflammatory benefits.

4. Mindful Meal Planning:

Tip: Plan meals with a balance of lean proteins, whole grains, and a variety of colorful fruits and vegetables for diverse nutrient intake.

5. Cooking with Coconut Oil:

Tip: Substitute coconut oil for other cooking oils; it adds a subtle tropical flavor and is suitable for moderate-heat cooking.

6. Quinoa Perfectly Cooked:

Tip: Rinse quinoa before cooking to remove bitterness. Use a 1:2 ratio of quinoa to water for perfectly fluffy results.

7. Fiber-Rich Choices:

Tip: Choose whole grains like brown rice and oats for their fiber content, promoting digestive health and stable blood sugar levels.

8. Sautéing Greens:

Tip: Quickly sauté leafy greens like spinach and kale with garlic and olive oil for some flavorful side dish rich in nutrients.

9. Roasting Vegetables:

Tip: Roast vegetables at high heat for a caramelized flavor. After tossing them in olive oil and adding some herbs, roast them till soft.

10. Marinades for Flavor:

Tip: Marinate proteins in herbs, citrus, and olive oil to infuse flavor and tenderize meats before cooking.

11. Balanced Smoothies:

Tip: Craft thyroid-friendly smoothies with berries, greens, a source of protein, and a liquid base like almond milk.

12. Mindful Snacking:

Tip: Opt for nutrient-dense snacks like nuts, seeds, and yogurt to keep energy levels stable between meals.

13. Hydration Habits:

Tip: Infuse water with herbs or fruits for a refreshing twist, encouraging hydration throughout the day.

14. Portion Control:

Tip: Be mindful of portion sizes to maintain a balanced diet. Use smaller plates to help manage portion control.

15. Batch Cooking for Convenience:

Tip: Prepare batches of thyroid-friendly meals in advance for convenient, healthy eating during busy times.

16. Colorful Plate Concept:

Tip: Aim for a colorful plate with a variety of fruits and vegetables to ensure a diverse range of nutrients.

17. Mindful Use of Sweeteners:

Tip: Use natural sweeteners like honey, maple syrup, or stevia in moderation to sweeten dishes and beverages.

18. Restful Eating Environment:

Tip: Create a calm eating environment. Sit down, savor each bite, and appreciate the nourishment your meal provides.

19. Adapt and Personalize:

Tip: Feel free to adapt recipes based on personal preferences and dietary needs. Cooking is an art; make it your own.

20. Enjoy the Process:

Tip: Cooking is an expression of self-care. Enjoy the process, experiment with flavors, and celebrate the nourishment you provide for your body.

Keep this quick reference guide handy in your kitchen for inspiration and guidance as you embark on your thyroid-friendly cooking journey. Happy and healthy cooking!